THE
SACRED BOOKS OF THE HINDUS

VOL. 15, PART 4

AMS PRESS
NEW YORK

THE
SACRED BOOKS OF THE HINDUS

Translated by various Sanskrit Scholars.

EDITED BY

Major B. D. BASU, I.M.S., (*Retired.*)

VOLUME XV.—PART IV.
THE YOGA SASTRA
INTRODUCTION TO YOGA PHILOSOPHY

PUBLISHED BY
SUDHINDRANÂTHA VASU
FROM THE PÂṆINI OFFICE, BHUVANEŚWARI ÂŚRAMA, BAHADURGANJ,
Allahabad
PRINTED BY APURVA KRISHNA BOSE AT THE INDIAN PRESS
1915

Library of Congress Cataloging in Publication Data

Vasu, Srisa Chandra, rai bahadur, 1861-1918?
An introduction to the Yoga philosophy.

Reprint of the 1915 ed. published by the Pāṇini Office,
Allahabad, which was issued as v. 15, pt. 4 of The Sacred
books of the Hindus, under the general title: Yoga sastra.
 1. Yoga. I. Title. II. Title: Yoga sastra. III. Series:
The Sacred books of the Hindus; v. 15, pt. 4.
B132.Y6V36 1974   181'.45   73-3806
ISBN 0-404-57838-1

Reprinted from the edition of 1915, Allahabad
First AMS edition published, 1974
Manufactured in the United States of America

International Standard Book Number:
Complete Set: 0-404-57800-4
Volume 15, pt. 4: 0-404-57838-1

AMS Press, INC.
New York, N.Y. 10003

AN INTRODUCTION
TO THE
YOGA PHILOSOPHY

BY

RAI BAHADUR ŚRIŚA CHANDRA VASU

PUBLISHED BY
THE PÂNINI OFFICE, BHUVANEŚWARI ÂSRAMA, BAHADURGANJ,
Allahabad
Printed by Apurva Krishna Bose, at the Indian Press
1915

TABLE OF CONTENTS

		Page.
Chapter	I	1
,,	II	7
,,	III	10
,,	IV	16
,,	V	20
,,	VI	23
,,	VII	29
,,	VIII	34
,,	IX	37
,,	X	49
,,	XI	51
,,	XII	54
Appendix	I	58
,,	II	64

FOREWORD.

Gheraṇḍa Sanhitâ is a Tântrika work, treating of Haṭha-Yoga. It consists of a dialogue between the sage Gheraṇḍa and an enquirer called Chaṇḍa Kâpâli. The book is divided into seven Lessons or Chapters and comprises, in all, some three hundred and fifty verses. It closely follows in the foot-steps of the famous treatise on Haṭha-Yoga, known as Haṭha-Yoga Pradîpikâ. In fact, a large number of verses of Gheraṇḍa Sanhitâ correspond *verbatim* with those of the Pradîpikâ. It may, therefore, be presumed that one has borrowed from the other, or both have drawn from a common source.

The book teaches Yoga under seven heads or Sâdhanas. The first gives directions for the purification of the Body (inside and out). The second relates to Postures, the third to Mudrâs, the fourth to Pratyâhâra, the fifth to Prâṇâyâma, the sixth to Dhyâna, and the seventh to Samâdhi. These are taught successively— a chapter being devoted to each (see Ch. I. v. 9-10-11).

The theory of Haṭha-Yoga, to put it broadly, is that concentration or Samâdhi can be attained by purification of the physical body and certain physical exercises. The relation between physical shell (ghaṭa) and mind is so complete and subtle, and their inter-action is so curious and so much enveloped in mystery, that it is not strange that Haṭha-Yogîs should have imagined that certain physical training will induce certain mental transformations.

Another explanation—and a later one—is that Haṭha-Yoga means the Yoga or union between ha (ह) and ṭha (ठ); the (ह) meaning the sun; and (ठ) the moon; or the union of the Prâṇa and the Apâna Vâyus. This is also a physical process carried to a higher plane.

The first question, which an unprejudiced enquirer will naturally put, after perusing this book, will be, are all these things possible ? and do these practices produce the result attributed to them ?

As to the possibility of these practices, there can be no doubt. They do not violate any anatomical or physiological facts. The practices, some of them at least, may appear revolting and

FOREWORD.

disgusting, but they are not *per se* impossible. Moreover, many of my readers may have come across persons who can practically illustrate these. Such persons are by no means rare in India. Every place of pilgrimage, such as Benares and Allahabad, contains several of them, in various stages of progress. My own Guru showed me and all his visitors at Allahabad and Meerut several of these processes, and taught some people how to do them themselves. The difficult processes, such as Vâri-Sâra (Ch. I. 17), Agni-Sâra (I. 20), Danda-Dhauti (I. 37), Vâsa-Dhauti (I. 40), &c., were all shown by him; so also the various Vastis, Neti, Âsanas, &c. Many of these may be classified as gymnastic exercises; their performers need not always be holy or saint-like personages. Several jugglers have been known to perform various Âsanas and Mudrâs, and earn their livelihood by showing them to the public. For persons whose muscles have become stiffened and the bones hardened by age, the acquirement of several of these postures, &c., is next to impossible; and it is better that they should not court failure or disappointment by attempting these at an advanced age. But Prânâyâma (regulation of breath), Dhâranâ and Dhyâna are possible for all.

As to the utility of these processes, genuine doubts may be entertained. Many of them may appear puerile, and, if not positively injurious, at least, useless. Although it is not possible within the short space at my command, to give the rationale of *all* these practices, and to justify them to a doubting public, I shall briefly illustrate the advantages of some of them. Thus, to begin with *Vâta-sâra* (I. 15). It is the process of filling the stomach with air, and expelling the wind through the posterior passage. The greatest duct or canal in the human body is the alimentary canal, beginning with the œsophagus (throat) and ending with the rectum. It is some twenty-six feet in length. This great drain contains all the rubbish of the body. Nature periodically cleanses it. Yoga practice makes that cleansing thorough and voluntary. If the cleansing is incomplete, then the fœtid matters putrify in the stomach and intestines, and generate noxious and deleterious gases which cause diseases. Now *Vâta-sâra* by passing a current of air through the canal, causes the oxidation of the fœtid products of the body; and thus conduces to health, and increases digestion. In fact, it gives a tone to the whole system. Similarly, *Vâri-sâra* is flushing the canal with water, instead of air. It thoroughly purges the whole canal; and does the same work as an aperient or a purgative, but with ten times more efficacy and without the injurious effects of these drugs. A person, knowing Vâtasâra and Vârisâra, stands in no need of purgatives: the same may be said of Bahiskrita Dhauti (I. 22). By Agnisâra (I. 20), the nerves and muscles of the stomach are brought under the control of volition; and by the gentle shaking of the stomach and the intestines, these organs lose their lethargy, and act with greater vigour. The washing taught in I. 23, 24, is a little dangerous, and may lead to prolapsus, and, a person who can do Vâri Sâra need not do this. The advantages of cleaning the teeth and the tongue are obvious, and, need not be dilated upon. The lengthening of the tongue (I. 32) is necessary for performing hybernation. In doing this, man but imitates the lower creation, like frogs, &c., who in hybernating turn their tongues upward, closing the respiratory passage. Perhaps, the most interesting of all Dhautis is the Vâsa-Dhauti (I. 41), which has led unobservant persons to the belief that the Yogîs can bring out the intestines by the mouth, wash them, and then swallowing them again place them in their proper position. This Dhauti is, however, a very simple process, and by so doing the mucus, phlegm, &c., adhering to the sides of the alimentary canal are removed. Water and air could not remove these viscid substances that stick to the sides of the canal.

The Neti, an easy process, clears the nostrils; and cures the tendency or predisposition to cold and catarrh. The Kapâlabhâti (I. 55) is a means of cleansing the frontal sinus, said to be the seat of Intelligence. This hollow cannot be directly reached from the outside, but by this process of Kapâlbhâti, the nerves surrounding it and spreading over the fore-head are brought into play and invigorated.

The various Âsanas taught in Chapter II are gymnastic exercises, good for general health and peace of mind, and calming of passions. The thirty-two Âsanas taught in this book are not all of equal efficacy or importance. Padmâsana is generally approved by all. The others may be practised occasionally for variation and recreation. Some of these postures help in checking animal passions by causing atrophy of the nerves of particular places. Others by straining and stretching of certain muscles create a pleasant sensation of strength and refreshment. The Âsanas are antidotes to the sedentary contemplation of Yoga—a habit

FOREWORD.

which may otherwise lead to mental hallucinations and nervous disorders.

The Mudrâs are similar to Âsanas in their action and efficacy. The gazing taught in some of these induces hypnotic sleep; and the Bandhas, by closing all the exits for air, produce a tension within the system, generating thereby a sort of electric current or force, called Kuṇdalinî Śakti. It is this Śakti which is the help-mate of the Yogîs in performing their wonders. The Khechari Mudrâ (III. 25-27) causes levitation of the body. That levitation is possible has now been established beyond doubt. What the particular conditions are, under which this takes place, has not yet been fully investigated by Western Science; but that the restraining of breath is one of these conditions may be said to be an undoubted truth. The Saktichâlana is a mysterious process, and until a person practically realises it, he can hardly believe it. The Mudrâs are mixed physical and mental processes, a bridge between Âsanas and Pratyâhâra.

The subject of Pratyâhâra is treated in Chapter IV in five ślokas. It is the process of restraining the mind from wandering, and restricting it to a fixed idea. All the five senses must be controlled, and they should not be allowed to divert the attention.

Prâṇâyâma is the Haṭha-Yoga *par excellence*. It is as dangerous when practised without the supervision of a competent teacher, as it is useful when practised under his supervision. To quote the words of a great authority on this subject: " By practising it according to rule, all diseases are destroyed ; but by doing so irregularly, all diseases are generated, such as hiccough, asthma, cough, head-ache, ear-ache, diseases of the eye, &c." A practical Guru is absolutely necessary to teach Prâṇâyâma: the directions given in this book are useful as subsidiary rules. Many mistakes and dangers will, however, be warded off by a strict adherence to these rules. The place—a small and solitary cell ; the time— spring and autumn ; the food—light and sâtwika ; these are some of the important preliminaries. Over-exertion, fasting, &c., should be avoided (V. 30.) This shows clearly that Haṭha-Yoga is not to be confounded with asceticism. It is far from that. As the training of an athlete is not asceticism ; so that of a Haṭha-Yogî is far from being so. True, celibacy is a necessary condition for both, but then that alone does not constitute asceticism. The directions regarding food are peculiar for the people of Bengal, the author of this treatise being apparently a Vaishṇava of Bengal. For other countries and persons, these directions may not be applicable in their entirety. But animal food, intoxicating liquors, tobacco, and drugs are strictly prohibited for all climes.

There are three parts of Prâṇâyâma:—Pûraka or drawing in of the breath; Kumbhaka or retaining the breath; and Rechaka or expelling the breath. The proportion of these should be 1 : 4 : 2, i.e., if Pûraka takes 12 seconds, Kumbhaka should be 48 seconds, and Rechaka 24 seconds. The ratio being kept the same, the period of retention, &c., may be increased *ad infinitum*. The beginner should proceed cautiously, and should not increase the periods of 16 : 64 : 32 seconds. He should carefully note the various mental and physical changes going on in his system while practising it. Perspiration should be wiped off with a dry towel: nor should he be afraid when he begins to feel a sort of quiver all over the body. Sometimes he may be jerked off his seat, sometimes he may involuntarily jump about the room like a frog. These should not frighten him. Sometimes there may be no physical manifestations, but mental reactions. He may hear noises, see visions, smell strange odours, or taste delightful delicacies. These are for the most part hallucinations, indicating an excited state of the nervous system. These will soon go off of themselves when not attended to. But flashes of truth will also illumine his heart now and then. Sometimes in the Chidâkâśa, he may see reflected distant scenes and events, thoughts of persons will become visible to him; and he himself may leave his body and be carried in space with incalculable velocity. All these symptoms accompany Prâṇâyâma. The Guru must always be near at hand to help and control; for otherwise insanity and not clairvoyance may be the outcome of all this. These are the results of higher stages of Prâṇâyâma. But every person may practise this for two or three minutes, and experience its beneficial results on his own body. Petty disorders, like head-ache, stomach-ache, chill before fever, weariness of body and mind will vanish instantaneously by performing two or three Kumbhakas. Some persons are born with the faculty of performing Prâṇâyâma—Swedenbourg was a living example of this in the West. All persons unconsciously perform Prâṇâyâma when absorbed in deep thinking.

The ten Vâyus (V. 60) are the various nervous forces or currents of the human body.

FOREWORD.

The various sorts of Kumbhakas taught in Chapter V do not require much elucidation. The Bhrâmarî Kumbhaka (V. 77), however, is a little peculiar. It leads one to hear the various sounds called Anâhata. These sounds are said to be caused within the body by the rushing of the blood through the arteries and veins. The fixing of mind on these sounds soon produces trance. Dhyâna and Samâdhi are purely mental processes. Fixity and one-pointedness of attention produce trance. The experiments of hypnotism prove this. To fix the mind on one idea produces exaltation of mental faculties.

S. C. V.

FOREWORD.

Śiva Saṃhitā is a Tântrika treatise on Yoga. It was translated by me as far back as 1884 and first published in the *Arya* of Lahore—a monthly journal conducted by the late Mr. R. C. Bary.

The mystic phraseology of the Tantras is very difficult to understand. My brother, Major B. D. Basu, I. M. S., the Editor of the Series of these Sacred Books of the Hindus, said in his Prize Essay on the Hindu System of Medicine published in the *Guy's Hospital Gazette* of London (1889), regarding the anatomy of the Tantras :—

"When these Tantras will be studied by oriental scholars, as closely as they have explored other branches of Sanskrit learning, the anatomical knowledge of the ancient Hindus shall be better known to the world ; " for, according to him, " better anatomy is given in the Tantras than in the medical works of the Hindus."

"From *Siva Saṃhitā* we learn that the Hindus were acquainted with the spinal-cord and the brain. They knew that the central nervous system is composed of grey and white matters. They discovered the central canal of the spinal-cord, and traced its connexion, through the fourth and third ventricles, with the lateral ventricles of the brain. They call it *Brahmarandhra*, or the dwelling-house of the human soul. The same Tantric work gives a description of the several ganglia and plexuses of the nervous system. The brain is said to be composed of *Chandrakalâ* or convolutions resembling half-moons."

In a paper on the Anatomy of the Tantras, originally published in the "Theosophist" for March 1888, Major Basu has tried to unravel the mystery of the Yogîs and Tântrists regarding the nerves and nerve-centres, and identify the *Nâdîs, Chakras,* and *Padmas.* The following is a reproduction from that paper :—

"The language of the Tantras being too allegorical and too mystical to be understood by the uninitiated, it is very difficult to identify the Nâdîs, the Chakras, and the Padmas described in them.

"However, some of the spots are easily identifiable from their simple and lucid description. Thus it is apparent that the "nectar-rayed moon" (*vide* Shiva Saṃhitâ, Ch. II, verse (6) is the underpart of the brain; that "Suṣumnâ" is the spinal cord; "Idâ" and "Pingalâ" are the left and right sympathetic cords respectively."

We shall try now to identify some of the nervous structures described in the Tantras:—

"Chitra."—From the description of this Nâdi in the Tantras (Shiva Saṃhitâ, Ch. II, verses 18-19), it may be identified with the grey matter of the spinal cord. For "in it is the subtlest" of all hollows called 'Brahmarandhra,' which is nothing else save the central canal of the spinal cord—a structure whose functions remain as yet to be discovered by the physiologists. The Tantrists appear to have traced its connection with the lateral ventricles of the brain. It has been considered by them to be the seat of the human soul. Even in these days, when it is no exaggeration to say that the Hindus have quite forgotten the scientific truths discovered by their ancestors, they point to the hollow space in the crown of the head (known as the anterior fontanalle) of the new-born child as the Brahmarandhra.

Every tyro in anatomy knows that this space contains the lateral ventricles of the brain.

The "Sacred Triveṇî" (Shiva Saṃhitâ, Ch. V, p. 52) is the spot in the medulla oblongata where the sympathetic cords join together or whence they take their origin. (*Vide* Ashby's Notes on Physiology,—Article Medulla Oblongata). The mystic Mount Kailâsa Shiva (Saṃhitâ, Ch. V, p. 154) is certainly the brain.

Padmas and Chakras.—Great difficulty arises in identifying these Padmas and Chakras. What are these structures one is tempted to ask? Are they real, or do they only exist in the imagination of the Tântrists? Though we are unable to satisfactorily identify them, we nevertheless believe that the Tântrists obtained their knowledge about them by dissection. These terms have been indefinitely used to designate two different nervous structures, *viz.*:—nervous plexuses and ganglia. But it may be questioned, how are we authorized to identify the Tântric Padmas and Chakras with either the ganglia or plexuses of the modern anatomists. Our reasons for doing so are the following:

1st.—The position of some of these Padmas and Chakras corresponds with that of the plexus or ganglion of the modern anatomists.

2nd.—These Chakras are said to be composed of petals designated by certain letters, which clearly point to either the nerves that go to form a ganglion or plexus, or the nerves distributed from such ganglion or plexus.

3rd.—Certain forces are said to be concentrated in these Chakras, thus identifying them with the plexuses or ganglia which the modern physiologists have proved to be "separate and independent nervous centres."

This Nâdî Suṣumnâ has six Padmas (Shiva Saṃhitâ, Ch. II, v, 27, p. 12), evidently signifying the six nervous plexuses formed by the spinal cord.

The description of the thousand-petalled lotus (Shiva Saṃhitâ, p. 51) shows it to be the medulla oblongata.

We proceed next to the identification of the famous six Chakras of the Tantras:—

i. *Mulâdhâra Chakra* (Shiva Saṃhitâ, p. 44) is the sacral plexus.

ii. *Swadhisthâna Chakra* (Shiva Saṃhitâ, p. 46). There can hardly be two opinions as to its being the prostatic plexus of the modern anatomists.

iii. *Manipur Chakra* (Shiva Saṃhitâ, p. 47) appears to be the epigastric plexus.

iv. *Anahat Chakra* (Shiva Saṃhitâ, p. 47) is the cardiac plexus.

v. *Viṣudha Chakra* (Shiva Saṃhitâ, p. 48) is either the laryngeal or pharyngeal plexus.

vi. *Ajnâ Chakra* (Shiva Saṃhitâ, p. 47) is the cavernous plexus.

We have very briefly hastened over the six Tântric Chakras. We see that these Chakras are the vital and important sympathetic plexuses, and preside over all the functions of organic life.

There can be little doubt that by the "contemplation" on these Chakras, one obtains psychic powers.

"Contemplation" leads to control over the functions of these Chakras or plexuses. "The intimate connection between the sympathetic nerves and the great viscera renders it highly probable that the sympathetic system has mainly to do with the organic functions. * * * The sympathetic is the system of organic life." When one gets control over the sympathetic nervous system, one is the master of one's body, one can die at will. The heart beats at his will. The lungs, the intestines, nay, all the different viscera of the body, carry on their allotted duties at the command of such a Yogî. Verily, verily that is the stage of Samâdhi.

Pratyâhâra must be clearly distinguished from Samâdhi. No more serious mistake, we think, can be committed than considering the hybernation of the reptiles and other animals as illustrating the Samâdhi stage of the Yogîs. The hybernation corresponds with the Pratyâhâra, and not the Samâdhi stage of Yoga. Pratyâhâra has been compared with the stage of insensibility produced by the administration of anæsthetics, *e.g.*, chloroform. But it is a well-known fact that the inhalation of chloroform has little perceptible effect upon the sympathetic nerves. The spiritual consciousness of man is intensified only when the functions of the organic life are brought under his control, and when he can modify and regulate the functions of the different viscera. We repeat that that is the stage of Samâdhi.

It behoves all students of Yoga and occultism then to gain a clear knowledge of these six Chakras, from the contemplation of which they can aspire to attain to the stage of Samâdhi."

In this connection, Dr. Brajendra Nath Seal's *Physical Sciences of the Hindus*, and the late Revd. Dr. Arthur Ewing's *The Hindu Conception of the Functions of Breath* may also be profitably consulted.

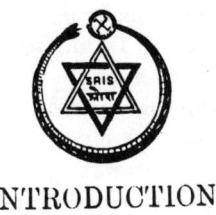

INTRODUCTION

TO

YOGA PHILOSOPHY.

CHAPTER I.

PRELIMINARY.

Yoga schittavritti-nirodhaḥ.

YOGA has been defined by Patanjali as the restraint of mental modifications (*Vrittis*). Any discussion of this subject, therefore, necessarily branches itself into three parts, *viz.*, (1) the *Mind*, (2) its modifications (3) and the *mode* of restraining them. No treatise on Yoga, can be complete, which does not enter into these questions. The nature of mind is the first thing which ought to be explained. It would embrace an enquiry into all those hypotheses which philosophers have formed about this entity. Is it immaterial and self-existent, or is it material and perishing, subject to dissolution with the body? Is it the same as spirit or is it apart from it? Is it merely a dream, a shadow, a reflection of the Supreme; or is it a separate and entire entity by itself? Such and many other questions of this nature must be answered before one has done away with the subject of Chitta (Mind). The second part consists of the enumeration, classification, and definitions of the various faculties of the mind. This part is generally free from controversy, as the faculties are facts more widely known and comprehended. This branch is what is known by the name of psychology. So far all the enquiry may be said to be preliminary :—but a preliminary absolutely necessary for the right understanding of the third part—*viz.*, *Nirodha* or restraint. That division contains all those various methods adopted by the ancients as well as the moderns for the concentration of the mind, which is the essence of Yoga. All the questions of diet, sleep, exercise, posture, &c., facilitating concentration naturally fall in that sub-division. A comparative view may also be taken in that as to the various means adopted by Yogis, saints, &c., for this purpose, as well as the contrivances used by the modern mystics to bring about this state of mind. In conclusion, we shall try to show what are the good results of Yoga, what are the spiritual faculties which it developes, what new channels for the acquisition of knowledge it opens, what new powers of work it creates and what a source of innocent, but sublime, happiness it forms for its votaries.

In this chapter we shall treat of two things:—*first*, the importance of the study of this Science, and *second*, the various objections which are generally raised against this subject.

The Importance of the study of this Science, and Objections.

The usefulness of this science as a means of mental culture has been often questioned. There are to be found many who even deny it the title of *science*. To their minds, the art and philosophy of Yoga have no better claims to be recognised as a branch of science, than alchemy or astrology. To them it is a dream of the poets, a hallucination of the enthusiasts. By what process of reasoning they have come to this conclusion, a conclusion contradicting almost all the religious as well as the philosophical convictions of the ancient and the modern times—is not very easy to decide. But so far as we can find, much of disbelief and scepticism is to be attributed to the ignorance of the real truths of Yoga. In India many understand by the word Yogi, those hideous specimens of humanity who parade through our streets bedaubed with dirt and ash,—frightening the children, and extorting money from timid and good-natured folk by threats, abuse or pertinacity of demand. Of course, all true Yogis renounce any fraternity with these. If these painted caricatures by any stretch of language can be called Yogis, surely their yoga (communion) is with ash and dirt, with mud and money.

There is another class of persons who have assumed this honored and sacred title, and who by their bigotry and ignorance have proved a great stumbling-block to the progress of this science. I mean the Hatha Yogis, those strange ascetics who by inflicting

CHAPTER I.

tortures and exquisite pains to their flesh, hope to liberate their spirits. Through a mistaken idea that mind and matter must necessarily be opposed to each other, they have evolved a philosophy of torture, whose fundamental doctrine seems to be :—the greater the power of spirit, the less you are pained by tortures. Some of these persons are seen sitting in the same posture for years together, their legs half paralysed by unuse ; some are seen with their hands upraised, which they never bring down, and which wither away and become dead stalks ; while others, in their supreme contempt of nature and everything natural, prefer to pass severe winter among snows, and the burning days of summer surrounded by fire. These persons by their misdirected energy and enthusiasm, have already done a good deal of mischief. They have engendered a belief in ordinary minds that Yoga is perfectly unattainable without austerities, that persons not prepared to fight with their physical nature such severe struggles as these Hatha Yogis, should never expect to make any spiritual progress.

Another, but far more gentle and rational, class of Yogis are those who might be called recluses. These persons are often very intelligent, and sometimes well-educated. But to us, these persons also seem to labor under a great error. By some false physical analogy they think that it is impossible to practise Yoga in household life, that to attain perfection in Yoga one must leave father and mother, wife and children, and run to deserts or high mountains. According to such, the *magnetic and mental atmosphere* (?) of cities and inhabited places is not favorable to spiritual culture, and only the deep solitudes of a cave or a desert are the best helps for Yoga. This belief that no householder can be a Yogi, is one tacitly believed in by our spiritual-minded Hindu brothers, who would no more think of practising Yoga without turning an ascetic than travelling to the moon. Nay, this belief is carried to an absurd extent by some sentimental Yogis of recluse type, who seriously maintain that the sacred and divine tie of marriage is an insuperable barrier in the path of a neophyte.

Looking on the disgusting spectacle of the ash-besmeared and lazy beggar, the horrible self-infictions of the Hatha Yogi, and inhuman apathy of the recluse, no wonder that many should think that Yoga is after all a great humbug, not worth the consideration of any sane man.

There is another class of objectors, who cannot bring their minds to believe the strange and weird powers which the practice of Yoga gives to its votary. Such are the scientists of our day—men of eminent learning and clear understanding, persons fitted by their education and pursuits for the proper investigation of such a complicated subject as Yoga. It is a pity that they should look with sublime disdain on the claims of Yoga to be recognised as a science. Powers such as those possessed by Śankarâcharya and Guru Nanak—foresight, transference of their *chitta* into other bodies, projecting their Kâma-Rûpa to distant places, healing the sick, &c., are so many stumbling-blocks to the modern scientist. Brought up in a school of severe reasoning, and strict and accurate observation and experiment, the scientist is unwilling to give his credence to the high pretensions of the Yogi without convincing proofs. Nor do we think that the demand is unnatural. But we had hoped, that his own good sense would have shown the scientist the futility of his objection. He ought to have known, that, while his science deals with things which can be perceived by the senses, and therefore can be demonstrated to all average humanity the very alphâbets of Yoga are Jivâtmâ and Paramâtmâ—things essentially supersensuous. In fact, there can be no analogy between the physical sciences and Yoga in this respect. The study of both the physical and mental sciences must, no doubt, be conducted through experiment and observation, but the objects of one are all tangible and outside of us, while the other has its materials in inward ideas and thoughts. Mathematics is perhaps the only science which can afford any slight analogy to Yoga. As it would be impossible for a common man· to understand the calculations by which an astronomer predicts an eclipse, unless he goes through years of mental training in Mathematics, so it is much more impossible to make ordinary scientific minds grasp the conclusions of Yoga, unless they are regularly initiated. As to the question why Yogis do not show *phenomena*, it might be answered in two ways. All Yogis have not the *power* of producing the visible manifestation of invisible forces. By far the great majority of Hindu Yogis practise it for the sake of spiritual development, and serenity and calmness of mind. *Siddhis* (psychic powers) are no ambition of their souls; they do not court them; nor are they elated if they produce some phenomena now and then. Their eyes bent upon *mokhsha*, these students of Yoga

CHAPTER I. 5

do not tarry in their course to pick up these baubles of *Siddhis*. Such persons, though never showing a single phenomenon in the course of their whole lives, intuitively produce conviction to our hearts by the purity, nay, almost the divinity of their lives. You can distinguish a real Yogi out of thousands, by that inexpressible serenity of his countenance, that nameless something about his look, voice and every movement of his limb, which are the invariable results of Sama and Dama—the control of mind and the control of senses. Wherever a Yogi goes, he carries happiness and purity with him. It is impossible to see a Yogi without being pleasantly influenced by him. He is the natural leader of humanity; his intense self-communion and concentration make him honored and respected, without any courting on his part. In short, a Yogi carries his credentials on his face. Such are the Yogis, with whom some of our readers might have had the pleasure of passing the happiest periods of their lives ; and if we are convinced of anything it is this that, be Yoga a delusion or hallucination, it *certainly* makes one *happy*.

That class of Yogis, who are called *Siddhas*, and who can produce phenomena, are extremely rare ; or at least they do not mingle much with mankind. But they are not so rare, as deligent search may not reveal them to the enquirer. It is these *Siddhas* only who can satisfy the experimental spirit of the scientist. It is they who at will can produce those psychical phenomena which cannot but convince the most confirmed sceptic. But for reasons, best known to them, *Siddhas* are always very reserved in displaying their powers to strangers. Long acquaintance and great intimacy with them can only break their reserve. Our scientific reader may very justly wonder at this, and think it rather inexplicable that persons knowing such a strange science should hesitate to establish its truth to the satisfaction of the outside world.

But this conduct of the *Siddhas* is not all so inexplicable and mysterious. Now, if we mistake not, a majority of the *Siddhas* are Hindus or belong to races nearly allied to Aryas. And Hindus, as is well-known, are the most jealous people on earth as regards their sciences. It is very hard to gain their confidence. The people of India have learned by sad experience that the only means of preserving their science and sacred scripture is in keeping them in strict secrecy. And it was no doubt a very safe means of preservation in olden times. We cannot but approve the policy of our ancestors in this respect. The world would not have appreciated the merits of our Sastras and Vedas had they been made public earlier. We are certain that many of our scientific works would not have been understood by the world two centuries before, even if made known to it. Even now, with all the advance which the sciences of language and grammar have made, we find how great injustice is done to our literature by occasional misinterpretation. It is only of late that our Panini's grammar has been acknowledged as the best treatise on the subject, nay, we may go even so far as to assert, that it is to the discovery of this book that we see all the attempts of modern Europe for the construction of a Universal Grammar. Well, when even Indian Pandits, who are anything but Yogis, were so very jealous with regard to those secular sciences, shall we blame the *Siddhas* that they are not more explicit and open. Surely they must have very good grounds for keeping their powers concealed from the gaze of the uninitiated profane. Surely we have no right to call them impostors and their science a moonshine, if they do not comply with our idle importunities. To sincere seekers after knowledge, to those who pant for spiritual regeneration, they are always accessible. They are ready to teach their science; they but seek persons who deserve that high gift. Where is the *adhikâri*, the truly qualified student. Where is he who has fitted himself by mental training, to pursue and understand the process or the processes, by which a Yogi acquires these mental powers? Where is the person who has the firmness of will, earnestness of purpose, doggedness of perseverance, by which alone success in any undertaking can be ensured? We know how few are the men who make any marked success in the ordinary human sciences. We do not see Newtons, Franklins, Tyndalls and Darwins everywhere, and must we expect to see Yogis and Siddhas made out of ordinary men—men whose spirituality is altogether dormant or dead.

CHAPTER II.

DEFINITIONS.

For ready reference, we here give the definitions of some of the important words. These definitions, as far as possible, are in the words of Patañjali.

1. *Yaga* is the restraining of the modifications of the thinking principle.

2. *Samádhi* (Meditation) is the intentness on a single point; or that state of knowledge in which the mind, having avoided the obstacles, is well fixed on, or confined to, one object only. It is a continual concentration of thought, by means of which all external objects, and even one's own individuality, are forgotten, and the mind fixed completely and immovably on the One Being.

3. *Samprajñáta-samádhi* (Meditation *with* distinct cognition) is that form of meditation which arises from the attendance of argumentation (*vitarka*), deliberation (*cichára*), beatitude (*ánanda*), and egotism (*asmita*).

4. *Asamprajñáta-samádhi* (Meditation *without* distinct recognition) is independent of any fresh antecedent, being in the shape of the self-reproduction of thought, after the departure of all objects.

5. *Abhyása* (Practice) is the repeated effort that the internal organ—Chitta—shall remain in its unmodified state, and in a firm position, without regard for the end in view, and perseveringly adhered to for a long time unintermittingly.

6. *Vairágya* (Indifference) is the consciousness of having overcome one's desires; this consciousness is of one who neither thirsts after the objects that are seen on earth, nor those that are heard of in the Scriptures.

7. *Vritti* (Modification of the internal organ) is the modification produced from either of the following five causes:—

   (*a*). *Pramána* (Evidence of right notion) is that which arises from perception, inference and testimony.

   (*b*). *Viparyáya* (Misconception) is incorrect notion, not staying in the proper form of that, in respect whereof the misconception is entertained.

8   YOGA PHILOSOPHY.

(c). *Vikalpa* (Doubt) ;—a notion devoid of a thing in reality corresponding thereto, following upon knowledge produced by words.

(d). *Nidrâ* (Sleep) depends on the conception of nothing.

(e). *Smriti* (Memory) is the not letting go of an object, of which the mind has been aware.

8. *Iswara* (Lord) is a particular Spirit (*Purusha*) untouched by troubles, works, fruits, or deserts, in whom the germ of the omniscient becomes infinite, who is the preceptor even of the first, for he is not limited by time, and whose name is Glory.

9. *Drashtâ* (Seer, soul) is a vision simply, though pure, looking directly ; it is the spectator merely through proximity. It is the mere thought. It alone is the experiencer.

10. *Avidyâ* (Ignorance) is the notion that the transitory, the impure, the evil and what is not-soul, are eternal, pure, joy and soul.

11. *Asmitâ* (Egotism) is the identifying of the power that sees with the power of seeing.

12. *Râga* (Desire) is that which dwells on pleasure : it is longing for the means of enjoyment.

13. *Dwesa* (Aversion) is that which dwells on pain.

14. *Abhinivesa* (Tenacity of life) is the attachment which every one feels naturally to the body, through dread of death.

15. *Yama* (Forbearance) consists of not killing, veracity, not stealing, continence, and not coveting.

16. *Niyama* (Religious observances) includes purification, contentment, austerity, inaudible mutterings, and persevering devotion to the Lord (Íswara).

17. *Âsana* (Posture) is the position which one sets himself to. It must be steady and pleasant.

18. *Prânâyâma* (Regulation of the breath) is the cutting short of the motion of inspiration and expiration.

19. *Pratyihâra* (Restraint) is the accommodation of the senses to the nature of the mind, in the absence of the concernment with each one's own object. It is the complete subjugation of the senses.

20. *Dhâranâ* (Attention) is the fixing of the internal organ (*Chitta*) to a place.

21. *Dhyâna* (Contemplation is the course of uniform (fixed only on one object) modification of knowledge at that place where the internal organ is fixed in Dhâranâ.

CHAPTER II.

22. *Samâdhi* (Modification) [see Def. 2] is the same contemplation or Dhyâna when it arises only about a material substance or object of sense, and therefore it is then like non-existence of itself and like ignorance.

23. *Sanyama* is the three, Dhâranâ, Dhyâna and Samâdhi, operating only on one object; or the technical name, for the above three taken together, is Sanyama.

24. *Antaraṅga* (Interior) is the name applied in Samprajñâta Samâdhi to the three Yogâṅgas: Dhâranâ, Dhyâna, and Samâdhi.

25. *Bahiraṅga* (Exterior) is the name applied in Samprajñâta Samâdhi to the five Yogâṅgas: Yama, Niyama, Âsana, Prâṇâyâma, and Pratyâhâra.

26. *Dharma* is that which follows upon, or has the properties in, the shape of Śânta (tranquil), Udita (risen), and Avyapradeṣ́ya (incapable of denomination). In other words, Dharma means the substance to which properties adhere.

27. *Siddhis* are the psychic faculties developed from the practice of Yoga.

CHAPTER III.

THE student of Yoga should, as far as possible, make up his mind what kind of Yoga method he is going to adopt. For, though the aim of the various systems of Yoga is the concentration of the mind, yet some are more difficult than the others, some lead to the attainment of Yoga earlier than the rest. Even there is difference in the capacity of student which ought to be taken into consideration. There cannot be given any hard and fast rule for all. All that can be done is to give the first principles, the primary truths, and leave the rest to the intelligent student to evolve out for himself. Difference of age, difference of education, religion, race and nationality, require different treatment from the hand of the master. Thus the methods of *Hatha* Yoga are such which an adult, after a certain age, can master with extreme difficulty, while to the plastic and supple limbs of a child or a boy of ten and twelve they are very easy of attainment. Similarly, a man whose mind is well cultivated with philosophy and poetry, whose fancy is vivid, whose imagination quick and creative, need not undergo any of those preliminary methods laid down in the treatises of Yoga for the development of imagination.

The period within which success in Yoga is acquired by the student also has proportional variation. To an energetic and enthusiastic nature success may crown his efforts very soon, while a dull person may pass years ere he understands the first principles of this mind-regulating philosophy. The treatises of Hindu Yoga are full of dissertations about the various kinds of persons fitted to acquire Yoga. In fact, the chapter on *adhikâris*, persons fitted for Yoga, forms generally the first in various systems of Yoga. The father of Yoga philosophy, Patañjali, disposes of this question with his characteristic brevity and universality by two *Sûtras* or aphorisms. That which puzzled the brains of the latter-day Yogis, and on which so much ingenuity has been mis-spent, has been compressed likewise by Patañjali within the narrow but all-embracing compass of two lines. Aphorism twenty-two, book first, enunciates:—" According to the nature of the methods—*the mild, the medium, and the transcendent*—adopted, the ascetics who adopt method, are of nine kinds."

CHAPTER III.

In accordance with this division, there are nine classes of followers of Yoga. In the mild variety there are three sub-divisions, and similarly with the medium and the transcendental methods. The following table shows the different kinds of followers of Yoga:—

Methods.	Classes of followers.		
	Mildly impetuous (*Mridu samvega*) simple or energetic.	Moderately impetuous (*Madhya samvega*) or impetuous.	Hotly impetuous (*Tivra samvega*) or hot.
Mild (*Mridu*) ...	1. Mildly energetic.	4. Mildly impetuous.	7. Mildly hot.
Medium (*Madhya*) ...	2. Middlingly energetic.	5. Middlingly impetuous.	8. Middlingly hot.
Transcendent (*Adhimátra*) ...	3. Extremely energetic.	6. Extremely impetuous.	9. Extremely hot.

Patañjali promises speedy success to him who is hotly impetuous and follows the transcendental method *i.e.*, he who comes under the ninth class of transcendent, hotly impetuous. Thus there is ample room for the student of Yoga Vidyâ to select from. He may follow the mild method, which is the lowest, or he may, if he can, take up the *Adhimátra* method. An explanation of these methods will be given further on. Now we shall speak of some of the preliminary things conducive to the concentration of mind, and thereby unfolding the spiritual powers latent in every human soul. In this chapter we intend to dwell on the following points—*food, dress, habits, and place.*

Patañjali in his aphorisms does not touch on any one of these points. He takes it for granted that the followers of Yoga have this requisite knowledge. In fact, the directions which the later authors on Yoga have given are such as are applicable not only exclusively to the student of occultism, but to every description of students. Nevertheless, we shall give here some short hints on this subject.

As regards dress, it must be borne in mind that the concentration is best facilitated when one is warmly dressed, and his attention is not distracted by the changes of weather. We think it highly unphilosophical to renounce all dress in the first stage of *Yoga abhyâsa*, as many of the Sâdhus are seen to do. Instead of helping in any way the fixing of attention, their naked bodies continually divert their thought. No doubt, the master Yogi needs no external help to protect his body from the inclemencies of the weather. He can throw around him an impenetrable veil of *âkâsa*, and defy the forces of nature; but what a master may do with impunity, can never be done by a neophyte without injury. The dress should not be too tight nor too loose, and, as far as possible, it should not be sewn by a tailor. If sewn-cloth cannot be dispensed with, let it be well purified of all foreign magnetism as far as possible. The clothes should be washed well every day by the student himself if possible, and it should be made a rule to change the lower garment at least once a day, and in no case to keep it on for two days without washing. The materials of which the dress of a Yogi should be made ought to be of non-conductors like silk, wool, cotton, &c.

As to the food most conducive to the spiritual and pschyic development, the authorities are unanimous in favor of a vegetarian diet, not that there were no Yogis who were meat-eaters, but it has been found by the concurrent experience of ages that meat, while it increases animal activity, decreases the power of concentration. All races of meat-eaters are physically active and strong, but the same cannot be said of their spiritual state. Animal passions and appetites are increased by the carnivorous diet, and the natural and constant restlessness of carnivorous animals is diametrically opposed to those conditions which favour quietness and abstraction. In recommending a vegetable diet for the student of the Yoga, we need not enforce our doctrine from consideration of occult philosophy, which he would not be in a position to understand were we to do so. In the very first stage of Yoga, *viz.*, *Yama*, the student is exhorted to practise *maitri*, universal kindness, and how can this be consistent with the cruel system of butchering innocent creatures for satisfaction of one's taste. We need not disprove the position of those who try to equivocate with their own conscience by saying that it is not they who kill but the butchers; for they ought to remember the aphorism of Patañjali, which says that—"' The things questionable,' *e.g.*, killing, stealing, &c., whether done, caused to be done, or *approved of*, whether resulting from covetousness, anger or delusion, whether slight, of intermediate character, or beyond measure, have no end of fruits in the shape of pain and ignorance." In fact, the vegetable

CHAPTER III.

world can supply all the constituents which a healthy human organism requres. As to the quality of food, the Yogis of India have all shown a great love for milk and rice. The chemical analysis of milk shows that it contains all ingredients which a human body requires, while rice is to be recommended chiefly on account of its containing proportionately smaller amount of stimulating nitrogenous matter which abounds so much in meats of every description. It must be all the while remembered, that the food above recommended is for Rishis and Yogis, and such persons whose habits are sedentary, and require intense mental abstraction; and therefore, this kind of diet has been called *satwa-guni-bhojan*. For warriors and mechanics employed in physical active duties of life *Rajoguni* food is the one to be recommended. The following verses of the Gita should also be remembered in this connection. Next as to the quality of food to be taken, let the student beware of gluttony; he should eat just enough for livelihood—for the support of life. But let him not at the same time starve himself to emaciation. It is desirable that he should eat less than usual, and rise from the table with appetite remaining than fully satisfied. Let him also decrease the quantity of food slowly, steadily, but imperceptibly. In fact, his progress through the several stages of Yoga will of itself tend towards decreasing the amount of food, but let him, nevertheless, help nature. In no case should the student of Yoga indulge in alcoholic or any other intoxicating drug or liquor, &c. The practices of some classes of inferior Yogis of stimulating psychic development by opium, bhang, charas and ganja, are to be strongly denounced by every sane and reasonable man: for these, though inducing momentary or temporary trance by their skilful administration, yet invariably are followed by terrible reaction, and make the divine temple of the soul a ruin for the vampires, spooks and elementals to take possession of and prey upon.

The student of Yoga, like his fellow-student of physical sciences, should cultivate regular habits. He should attend to all the rules of health and sanitation. Early rising and the Yoga abhyâsa for an hour or so before sunrise have been often recommended. The would-be Yogi must attend to the purity of the body as well as the soul. Let him bathe twice daily, in the morning and evening, and, if his constitution would allow, with cold water, at all seasons of the year. Several Yogis of the Sikh school, maintain that the keeping of long hair, by preserving the animal electricity, facilitates Yoga. And in truth the majority of Saints, Rishis, and Prophets are generally represented with flowing hair. The Yogi should choose a retired and unfrequented spot for practising Yoga. A league or two away from the bustle of active life, let the contemplative student select his retreat. The place should be such as to call up pure and divine thought. But it is also possible for a student to live in the city and aquire Yoga. And, as the majority of our readers, I fear, are *Grihastas*, householders, and family-men, let them, therefore, set apart a room in their house sacred for meditation. Let it never be entered by anybody and every-body; and it should be so situated or constructed as effectually to exclude all outside noise and commotion. If he likes he may burn incense, like *dhoop*, &c., to make the atmosphere of the room sweet and agreeable. The Buddhist scriptures enjoin the following particulars about the choice of place by the ascetic :—" It is a place where no business is transacted, and where there are no contentions or disputes. There are three descriptions of such places : (1) in some deep mountain ravine, remote from human intercourse ; (2) in some forest resort (Aranya), at least a mile or two from a village, so as to be removed from any sound of worldly business or contention ; (3) in a spot at a distance from a place where laymen live, in the midst of a quiet Sangharama " This precept of the Buddhistic school is, however, practicable only to the ascetic who has renounced all the concerns of the world. But as we tried to show in our preliminary remarks, Yoga is not meant only for the ascetic, but is a common heritage of the *Grihasta* and *Sanyâsi*, rich and poor

Next as to the time of practising Yoga. Every person who has a sound mind and a healthy body is capable of attaining Yoga. The training should be begun as early in life as possible. In old age, when the habits are crystallized into second nature, it becomes almost impossible for the student to shake off the old Adam and to turn over a new page in life. Our countrymen have imbibed certain mistaken notions as to the proper age when Yoga should be begun. They assert that great kings, &c., practised Yoga towards the close of their lives when they had completed their wordly career, had children and grand-children, and had been satiated by satisfying all their carnal appetites. The great poet, Kâlidâsa, in his *Raghuvansa* says of the kings of the solar dynasty :—*Yogenânte tanu tyajâm*, *i.e.*, they (the kings) left their bodies (*i. e.*, died) by practising Yoga. But it must be remembered that Janaka also was a great king and a great Yogi, too; similarly, Dhruva and Prahláda were children when they had acquired great Yogic powers. It should also be borne in mind that the very training of all our kings and great men, though not strictly Yogic, was yet conducive to spiritual development. Yoga should be begun as soon as the child reaches years of discretion. The proper time of *abhyâsa* is morning, and, according to Mahomedan Sufis, midnight. It should be practised with empty stomach, but seldom after a meal.

The student should do well not to sleep more than six hours. Sleep is overpowering of the mind by *Tamo-Guna*. The Budhistic saying is, "too much sleep destroys all religious merits. By not yielding to the influences of sloth, either one night or two, rejecting and not listening to its bewitchments, the life is cleansed and there is nothing further to attain." We do not recommend such an extreme course, but we can assure him there is much truth in the above saying, and that he will do well if he fasts twice or thrice a month, and observes vigils occasionally.

There is another advice of the Buddhists which we quote here for our readers:—" Care must be taken that no violent exertion be used previous to entering on the exercise of meditation, lest the breath should be agitated and the mind in consequence unsettled."

CHAPTER IV.

In our last chapter we dealt with some of the physical qualifications of a student of this science. In the present chapter we shall briefly glance over some features of the mental training indispensably necessary to him, as it paves the way to the final goal, the concentration of the mind.

There are certain spiritual obstacles which the Yogi will find in the very beginning of his career, and which, if not timely guarded by the warning voice of his *guru*, are sure to cause miserable shipwreck in his hopes of future progress. A would-be Yogi tries to separate, by the force of concentration, his soul from the body; and in that emancipated state he enjoys the blissful pleasure of the company of spirits more or less elevated in the scale of advancement. By the very act of being thus enabled to roam free through the eternity of time and space, cutting off the shackle of the material body, he incurs new dangers to which he was not liable before ;—dangers arising from the jealousy of *Devatás* presiding over the various elements. Those acquainted with the true significance of the sacred Puránás will readily conceive our meaning. The *Devatás*, Indra, &c., who so often tempt the sage and anchorite, are, none, if rightly understood, but the spirits of fire, air and water. They are intelligent entities, with tremendous powers, and the only mode of overcoming them lies through the path of Yoga. The student of Yoga will, therefore, find himself surrounded by these influences, which, though invisible, nevertheless act very powerfully. These elementals constantly whisper strange suggestions and distract thoughts, in order to withdraw him from contemplation, but he should not listen to those promptings of his "imagination." No blame, however, should be attached to the Devas for so doing. They have their scope and jurisdiction, and test the student from time to time. They are the true soul-examiners. Happy the man who has such " temptations " thrown in his path, for that is the sure sign that he is making progress and has attracted the attention of these Higher beings. Some of these obstacles are now being mentioned in detail.

The first and foremost temptation which the student meets with is from his passion, particularly from that of lust. Sexual desires

CHAPTER IV. 17

will overcome him with irresistible force, vague yearnings will torture his every-day existence, and they will be the more powerful, the more idle he is. The common proverb, that Satan finds some mischief for idle hands to do, is nowhere so well illustrated as in the case of the young Yogi. His sedantary habits, if not well regulated, peculiarly pre-dispose him to these temptations, and it is to guard against them that such minute details are often given about food, regimen, posture, &c. To prevent distraction proceeding from this cause, the Sikh Guru Arjun advised his *chelas* to be married. He knew that, though Yoga, like poetry, is a very jealous mistress, and that for the highest development of psychic powers, celibacy, or, at least moderation, was an important condition, still he had well probed the depth of the human heart, and by his own example of married life showed that it is compatible with Yogic education.

Patañjali enumerates the following nine obstacles:—Sickness, langour, doubt, carelessness, laziness, addiction to objects of senses, erroneous perception, failure to attain any stage of abstraction, and instability in it when attained. These are the primary distractions; there is yet another class which may be called secondary, *viz.*, grief, distress, trembling and sighing. The method of overcoming these obstacles is through *abhyása* and *Vairágya*. In fact, *Vairágya* (indifference) will be of the greatest help to the student. If he is grieved at the death of a dear friend, let him betake to *Vairágya*, take shelter under its shade and hear its sweet and solemn admonitions, saying—"nothing is permanent in this transitory world." If suffering from the excruciating pains of sickness and disease, let him resort to this never-failing doctor *Vairágya*, and his pains will vanish. Martyrs have died on the stake without showing the slightest sign of pain, though their flesh was torn from the body by inches. What was it that supported them through this horrible trial of the physical nature? Their mind no doubt. Is it then too much to expect from the aspirant that he should conquer his nerve-life by the indomitable strength of *Vairágya*? Truly, there lie hid innumerable wonderful potencies under the covering of *Vairágya*! Disease, distress, grief, nay, all obstacles, vanish like mist before the burning rays of *Vairágya*. Learn, therefore, betimes to practise this virtue.

Besides *Vairágya*, there are enumerated by Patañjali some five or six other methods of eliminating the evil consequences of the above-mentioned obstacles. Firstly, by profound devotedness towards the Lord Iśwara. We have already defined the term Iśwara. This devotedness to God is an easy method of attaining Yoga. Those who adopt this system are called followers of Bhakti-márga. The majority of the Aryans of India now know no other method than this. It is very popular with the masses; and that it is a very successful method is proved beyond doubt by the lives of the religious saints and fakirs who perform wonders by their faith in the Lord God. By devotedness is not to be understood the hypocritical system of prayers which passes by that name. It must be entire resignation to God, accompanied with intense love. It must be the forgetfulness of self,—living in the Lord. We must worship the Lord, not only with flowers and incense, but with "repeating His name and reflecting on its signification." He has got many names amongst different nations, but the Hindus have assigned most mystical powers to the word "Om." This word is called pranava (glory), and its repetition is enjoined as a help to concentration. The Mahomedans use Alla-hu, the Sikhs Váh Guru the Buddhists Om mani padme hum, the Jews Jah-ve. The proper pronunciation of the pranava and reflecting on its signification, brings with it the knowledge of the Lord.

The second method of over-powering these obstacles is "Dwelling upon one truth." We must fix our attention again and again upon some one accepted truth; we must concentrate our mind upon one point, and allow it under no circumstance to wander from it. Another method is "through the practising of benevolence, tenderness, complacency, and disregard towards objects of happiness, grief, virtue and vice." Benevolence but half represents the meaning of the original Sanskrit word Maitri. It is a term of larger signification than even charity. It is good-heartedness and love confined not within the limited circle of humanity, but extending to all animate creation, friendliness towards the creatures of God,—something more than philanthropy. 'Tenderness' is showing compassion to the unfortunate, the wretched and the poor: while "complacency" is that state of sympathy which feels joy in the happiness of a fellow-creature. The whole essence of this method may be summed up in the comprehensive word—"Sympathy,"—universal sympathy, sympathy for the animate and inanimate creation. The fourth expedient of combating mental distraction is "by forcibly restraining the breath," i.e.,

CHAPTER IV.

Prânâyama. We will treat of it in detail in the next chapter. The fifth method mentioned by Patanjali is "by fixing the attention on any object cognizable through the senses." The student may fix his attention on the tip of the nose, the centre of the tongue, &c. Another method is "by fixing the attention on a luminous object." * This is more active, and produces, in certain constitutions, the trance state sooner than other methods. Placing a luminous object a yard or so at a distance, and looking at it steadily for some minutes, keeping the head all the while at an angle of 45° will almost induce hypnotic trance. The mystic needs no external luminous object to fix his eyes upon : he sees a pure steady light in the "lotus of his heart." The seventh means of combating distraction is "by fixing the mind on some person whose life is holy and devoid of passion." This method is in great favor with the Jainas and Buddhists. Many followers of those persuasions keep the images of their *gurus* in their houses, and in ordinary parlance are said to worship them, and are consequently branded by ignorant bigots as idolaters and hero-worshippers ; but to those who know rightly, they do no such thing ; they only contemplate the image of their *guru*, as a means of facilitating mental concentration.

The eighth method of Patañjali is :—

"By dwelling on knowledge that presents itself in transition from waking to dream or to sleep." This transition state is a natural state of Yoga. When passing from the state of waking to that of dream, the mind passes through a zero point. Similarly when passing from the state of dream to that of dreamless sleep. These zero points of consciousness are the natural states of *samâdhi* or concentration. Hypnopompic and hypnogogic are the modern names given to some of these states. Just before falling into sleep or coming out of sleep, wonderful pictures pass before mind's eyes. Fixing attention on these is helpful.

"*Concentration of the mind may be effected by pondering on anything that one approves.*" Different persons have different temperaments, and no hard and fast rule can be laid down for this purpose to fit them all. Thus the Tantriks have their own ways, the Sufis their own, and the Buddhists their particular system, and so also the mystic Christians.

---
* This method is called Braidism.

CHAPTER V.

In the last chapter we dwelt on the theoretical side of the question of steadying the mental function; in the present, we shall consider the practical means of bringing it about. Practically the subject consists of three divisions - (1) *tapa* (reflection; as well as mortification of the flesh); (2) *sradhyâya* (repeating of some sacred formula or mantras); and (3) *pranidhâna* (resignation or consigning unto the Lord all the *fruits* of one's works, without expecting any reward, here or hereafter.)

By this practice, different kinds of afflictions, such as ignorance, egotism, desire, aversion and tenacity to mundane existence, are removed. Ignorance is in fact the parent of all the rest, and when that is removed, the extinction of others is but a matter of time, and comparatively easy. We have defined them before, and we may say that they can be got rid of by meditation. Our *karma* owes its origin to these afflictions, which result in constant re-births. The fruits of the *karma* are received sometimes in this life, but generally in the next. The *karma* is the root, while the fruits which it produces are—(*a*) rank (raised or lowered such as that of angel, planetary spirit, man, elemantal, bird or beast); (*b*) years (duration in which the spirit is confined in body); (*c*) enjoyment (sensation or experience of pleasure and pain). The fruits of good *karma* are joyful, and of the vicious painful. Even this suffering and enjoyment must be taken in their relative signification, for to a truly discriminating philosopher *all* is grief. For what ordinary men consider pleasure is but a modification of grief,—for it is never lasting. Being but transitory, its absence causes pain. The more we enjoy, the more we become miserable, for, with the increment of the sources and objects of pleasure, our desires and wants also increase, and disappointment at the non-attainment of those wants. Real wisdom does not consist in increasing our wants, which the civilization of the present age has been at pains to multiply, but in the opposite direction. The fewer our wants, the happier we shall ultimately be.

Vexation and anxiety will ever be the lot of those who hunt after pleasure and temporal happiness, instead of philosophy and quietism. Let it be clearly realised by the student of Yoga that the great secret of *true* happiness consists in considering *all* objects as sources of grief. It is through ignorance that man thinks one thing pleasant and another painful; but let the curtain of *Avidyâ* be removed from his mind, and he will see that all objects are equally painful or pleasant, in fact, he will be indifferent to them all. Let a wise man, therefore, shun the pain which has not yet come, and the fear of future pain will hold him back from present pleasure: for he will understand that every pleasure has in it the nidus of pain. If you ask, whence is this evil which we see in this world, we reply that there is no such thing as evil; what appears so is due to *Avidyâ*. To the philosopher who has attained right knowledge, all is equal. The origin of evil lies in the relationship of the *seer* with the *seen*, *soul* with *non-soul*, *spirit* with *nature* (material), *experiencer* with the *experienced*. The idea that soul is different from nature is the cause of all evil:—It arises from confounding the attributes with their substratum or receptacle in which they adhere. All grief vanishes when the Yogi clearly understands the grand truth that matter exists but through the spirit; that nature has no real existence of its own, but has its being through the entity, spirit—in fact, matter is dependent on spirit for its existence, and not the latter on the former. Or as Patañjali has it:—" For the sake of it (soul) alone is the entity of the visible (matter)." The soul reaches the state of *kairalyam* isolation when it separates itself from matter and dwells in its own pure light. To such a soul, even on earth, mundane existence ceases to have any tangible reality, though to others who have not elevated themselves by this consideration, the world might possess an existence, too gross to be safely ignored.

But let us not be understood from the foregoing remarks that we recommend anything like misanthropic asceticism and inhuman self-mortification. These practices we have all along strongly denounced, and we think it our duty to enter our protest against them again in this place. Let a Yogi be *unselfish*, but not inhuman; let him search real happiness in his soul, and not in the world; let him move through the scenes and vicissitudes of life as a calm witness (intelligence), seeing all, feeling all, enjoying all, neither absorbed in any one, nor engrossed by them. To quote an old maxim—let him be a pearly liquid drop on a lotus-leaf, moving on it, but not adhering to it, ever keeping his soul free from all selfish anxieties and cares of the world, but taking nevertheless active and earnest interest in the welfare of humanity. Let him conquer sorrow, grief and pain by contemplating upon the following sublime words of one of the brightest—if not the brightest—gem of humanity, Lord Buddha:—

"The first truth is of *sorrow*. Be not mocked!
Life which ye prize is long-drawn agony:
Only its pains abide; its pleasures are
Like birds which light and fly.

"The second truth is *sorrow's cause*. What grief
Springs of itself and springs not of desire?
Senses and things perceived mingle and light
Passion's quick spark of fire.
The third is *sorrows's ceasing*. This is peace
To conquer love of self and lust of life,
To tear deep-rooted passion from the breast,
To still the inward strife;
For love to clasp eternal beauty close;
For glory to be Lord of self, for pleasure
To live beyond the gods; for countless wealth,
To lay up lasting treasure.
Of perfect service rendered, duties done,
In charity, soft speech, and stainless days,
The riches shall not fade away in life,
Nor any death dispraise.

"Then sorrow ends, for life and death have ceased,
How should lamps flicker when their oil is spent?
The old sad count is clear, the new is clean,
Thus hath a man content."
                    Arnold's *Light of Asia*.

CHAPTER VI.

"The fourth truth is *the way*. It openeth wide,
Plain for all feet to tread, easy and near,
The noble eight-fold path, it goeth straight
To peace and refuge, Hear!"*

Now we enter upon the best known and most practical part of Yoga, *viz.*, *Yama, Niyama, Âsana, Pranayâma, Pratyahâra, Dhâranâ, Dhyâna* and *Samâdhi*. The first five belong to the *Bahiranga, i.e.*, external Yoga, while the latter three to internal Yoga. These eight steps lead to the final goal of *Kaivalyam* or *isolation*, otherwise called emancipation, *Mokhsha* or *Nirvâna*.

1.—*Yama*.

Yama consists of five parts, and is the universal duty of all. It enjoins *ahinsâ* (not-killing), *satya* (truth), *asteya* (not stealing), *Brahmacharya* (continence, and perfect chastity), *aparigraha* (not coveting). It is a duty incumbent on all persons, whatever be their rank, nationality or country. It forms the first chapter of the universal code of morality. Almost all the evils of the world may be traced, directly or indirectly, to a breach of some one of these laws. Strict observance of these rules brings with it its own reward. However, we shall mention some of the perfections which a Yogi acquires, who adheres firmly to them. When a Yogi becomes completely harmless and has no *hinsâ* whatever, then in his presence all ferocious animals forget their ferocity, none of them dare injure him, nor cause harm to each other while under his influence. When a Yogi becomes a perfect lover of truth, and practises always veracity, he amasses a store of good *karma* without performing the usual sacrifices, alms, &c. When his abstinence from theft is complete, all jewels of the earth, in whatever quarter they may be hid, come to him unasked, that is, he can command wealth if he leaves off totally the desire of wealth. If he practises perfect *Brahmacharya*, he gains strength. And it is but reasonable that it should be so: for every act of unchastity is destructive to self and power. If his uncovetousness is complete, he regains the knowledge of all his former states of existence. That this should be so is a

---

* Arnold's *Light of Asia*.

mystery apparently. But the word covetousness should be taken in its largest sense, i.e., the soul should not covet the body, which is its tabernacle and temporary home; and thus when it becomes free from the body by discarding it, it gains the knowledge of its past lives and deaths, and of the bodies which it had once filled. Of course virtue must be practised for its own sake without looking to any ulterior end, but in the economy of nature good acts are ever followed by good fruits. Nor must the above perfections, resulting from the practice of *Yama*, be regarded as fictitious and imaginary. Lives of holy Rishis and saints, of every country and age, bear ample testimony to the truth of this doctrine. A person who loves all creatures, whose soul is in sympathy with all animate creation, emits a magnetic aura of great potentiality, and every creature, however ferocious, must feel its influence. The most ferocious brute dares not lift its eyes in his presence, for the law of sympathy requires it so. Thus *ahinsâ* made Pythagoras and Buddha tamers of the brute creation. We read in Manu:—" He who injures no animated creature shall attain without hardship whatever he thinks of, whatever he strives for, whatever he fixes his mind on."

Similarly, we can understand that a person who practises veracity acquires a store of good *karmas*, though he may not perform a single *yajna*. Of all virtues, truth is the most divine, and one who adheres to it has no need of sacrifices and ablutions. He will never do wrong or injustice, and thus, though not performing *karma*, will get its fruits.

"When abstinence from theft is complete, all jewels come near him." Let it not be thought to be an inducement for not stealing; noncommission of theft is after all not a great virtue. But what the author means is probably this, that a Yogi should not even entertain the thought of possessing, by unlawful means, the property of another. The word *steya*, translated into theft, includes fraud, misrepresentation, cheating, and even adultery; for wife is said to be the property of her husband.

Similarly, that the practice of *Brahmacharya* (chastity) should give strength, is very clear. There is a class of medical men who think total abstinence from sexual intercourse is productive of as injurious results as excessive venereal or sexual indulgence. They argue that every organ must have its normal and healthy use, while unuse must result in the atrophy of that part. From considerations

CHAPTER VI.

like these they assert that celibacy is prejudicial to longevity, *Brahmacharya* is a violation of the creative and reproductive law of nature. There is much truth in these remarks; but do we not think that celibacy is meant by the word *Brahmacharya*? Though for our own part, we believe celibacy unnatural, yet we are not prepared to admit that it is injurious to longevity. We have seen perfect celibates enjoying the best health possible, and attaining to old age. However, we think with Manu that it is not total abstinence only which constitutes *Brahmacharya*, but moderation. "He who abstains from conjugal embraces on the six reprehended nights and on eight others, is equal in chastity to a Brahmachâri, in whichever of the two next orders he may live." Nor is total abstinence a *sine quâ non* of *Yoga*. There have been Hindus, Sikhs, Mahomedans, &c., who were married men, with wives and children, and still good Yogis. The best of them, in fact the teacher and discoverer of Yoga, the very ideal of a Yogi—stands the sublime picture of Siva. Students of the Indian Yoga worship Him as the *param guru*—the great teacher—and a large class of people contemplate nothing but his attributes in their *Dhyâna*. He, the founder and discoverer of this spiritual science, showed by his life that marriage, instead of being an obstacle in the path of spiritual enlightenment, positively facilitates the development. He is represented not only as a Yogi-râja, but the most loving of husbands and the kindest of fathers. Therefore, it is but reasonable to conclude that, by *Brahmacharya* the author Patañjali, does not mean celibacy, but continence.

The fifth part of *Yama* is "*non-coveting*." Its fruit is the knowledge of past lives. It has been already explained what is meant by *aparigraha*, whose English equivalent, in the absence of anything better, we have given as above. It is that state in which the soul does not desire to have anything which is not its own; and, as body is no part of the soul, but is only a temporary house in which the soul resides, or rather a wonderful instrument on which the soul plays, a love therefore of body is a love of a thing which is not-soul, and, therefore, amounts to *parigraha*, or covetousness. That *aparigraha* produces knowledge of past existences, establishes, through implication, a much contested point in metaphysics, *viz.*, that the human soul has to pass through successive stages before it becomes human. Many of us have been nurtured in the belief that the soul is created with the body, and thus, though it has a beginning, it is nevertheless eternal. The position taken up by Patañjali and almost every school of Indian philosophy is that, not only the soul has no end, but it has no beginning as well. It had experienced many existences before it became human. The Yogi knows his past lives, which an ordinary man does not. But the question arises—did our souls exist before as human, or had it any other body, e.g., of the beast or the brute? The principle of progress, as evidenced throughout the works of nature, proves to demonstration that the human soul has become so by passing through *lower* stages of existence,—stages of mineral, vegetable, and animal—and that this progress is in a spiral line, and not in a circle. The theory of transmigration is reasonable only in so far as it propounds the doctrine of previous and subsequent existences, but it is grossly in error if it inculcates that man, however depraved, will ever revert to a brute or beast again. Those who quote Patañjali in support of the latter doctrine, seem not to have grasped the full spirit of his philosophy. He, no doubt, believes in the previous existences of soul, but there is no mention in his writings of this retrogression. The soul of a beast after a course of ages may become human; but once human, it can, under no ordinary circumstances, ever revert to beasthood. Taking it then as reasonable that man had previous existences in the shape of lower animals, the next difficulty that arises is, how does one gain back the reminiscences of those long forgotten ages by simply non-coveting of his body. To understand this properly, the enquirer should realise that there is no past, present or future in eternity; nothing perhaps explains it so clearly as the phenomena of light. Suppose two persons, A and B, quarrel in a dark room, and A strikes down B dead. Just at the moment when B falls, a light is brought into the room, when a third person, C, whom we suppose to be standing near the door of the room, will see B fall just actually at the very moment when B fell. How did he see it? Because the light, which was introduced into the room, carried with it the picture of B from the room into the eye of C standing outside. Suppose the distance from B to the eye of C to be 18 feet, the time which light will take to travel from B to C will be so very inappreciable that we may call it instantaneous. But suppose C is situated at the distance of 180,000,000 miles instead of 18 feet, now the light which will reach his eyes will do so, ten seconds after it was brought into the room, and C will see B falling ten seconds

CHAPTER VI.

after the actual event. Again, suppose C is standing on the star named Serius, and looking towards the room in which A and B fight. Now, astronomers have calculated that light takes about three years to travel from Serius to the earth, and *vice versa*. So C will see B falling some three years after the event, *i.e.*, if B was killed in 1880, C will see it in 1883. Thus, what passed with us three years ago, will be present to C. To take another example :— Suppose we wish to see the Durbar of Delhi which took place in 1911, in the month of January. On our earth it is past three years. If we go to the distance of Serius, and then look towards the spot on the earth where Delhi is, we shall see the whole Durbar passing before our sight. In fact, light carries for ever through space the pictures of things, and it is a calculation involving simple multiplication to find out at what distance a particular picture will be found at a particular time. The original may have perished long ago, but its picture is retained for eternity in light. Under certain circumstances, the picture of the past is possible to be seen on this earth. Taking the above example of the Durbar, light travelled from the Earth to the Serius in three years, and reached that star in 1914 : if this light be reflected from it by some polished surface back towards the earth three years after 1911, that is, in 1914, so that even in this earth, if we will know the proper ray and catch it, we shall see the Durbar of Delhi three years after it actually took place. Thus by reading the pictures in the *ákás* (other), one can know the past. Physical science may perhaps discover some day the means of developing these pictures impressed in the *ákás* ; but spiritual science has already attained it. Psychometry is a standing proof of this. And the means for attaining this end, as proposed by Yoga, is "covet not the body." Let the human soul free itself from this mortal coil, this prison-house of body, and in its *Liṅga sarîra* (the etherial duplicate), it will be enabled as easily to read pictures impressed in ether, as in its material body it perceives phenomena.

Thus we have enumerated all the five parts of *yama*. They have been very aptly called the *mahâ vratas* or the great duties. These *vratas* must have precedence over all other *vratas*. Those ceremonies which we now-a-days call *vratas*, such as fasting on the eleventh day of the moon, giving alms to Brahmans, &c., are all inferior to them. One who does not kill the most insignificant of the living creatures of God, commits no theft, violates not the law of chastity, tells no falsehood, and covets not anything of the world, needs not perform any other *vrata* or ceremony. He needs not the guidance of priests, for he is a guide to himself. He may defy all the opposition of the ignorant of the age, and bravely go on in his path of duty.

CHAPTER VII.

2.—*Niyama*.

THE second part of Yoga is *niyama* or sacred observances. It consists of five parts, *viz.*, (1) *śaucha* (purification), (2) *santoṣa* (contentment), (3) *tapa* (austerity), (4) *swadhyáya* (inaudible and incessant repetition of the word), and (5) *Iśwara-pranidhána* (persevering devotion to the Lord). These form the second step of the ladder of Yoga. When one has got complete mastery in the practice of the five *mahávratas*, then one should turn one's attention towards gaining perfection in these five sacred observances. They all relate to practices calculated to bring about a calm state of mind, and thereby prepare it for concentration.

We shall now enumerate the fruits of this five-fold observance. The result of purification, which means mental as well as bodily purification (*a*) is two-fold :—" It produces a loathing for one's own members and non-intercourse with others, and (*b*) produces the purity in the quality of goodness, complacency, intentness, subjugation of the senses, and fitness for beholding the soul." A clean body can only contain a pure soul, and if the bodily tabernacle be kept unclean and impure, the indwelling soul receives the taint. We cannot believe that a person who swelters in impurities of the flesh can possess a pure soul. A filthy body must have a filthy tenant. It is from this consideration that we condemn those Haṭha Yogis, who live a filthy physical life, whose bodies smell of odours inexpressible, and many of whom glory in the command over their nerves, as expressed in swallowing filth and ordure of every kind. Such practices are simply disgusting and not countenanced by true Yoga. Purification of the body produces mental purification, which in itself is not a small gain. But besides that, it produces, as said above, a loathing for one's own members and that of others too. When we clearly see before our mental sight what a sack of foulness and filth our body is, what a veritable dung-hill of nuisance is contained within it, we cannot but feel disgusted with it, and begin to love our bodies less and our souls more. This purification also detaches our souls from the 'love of women and beautiful faces. It at once reminds us that physical beauty is but a painted sepulchre, containing within it abominations, and that our souls should not be ensnared in the meshes of outward charms, but piercing through the fleshy curtain, look into the soul within and fall in love with that, if it be beautiful. Beautiful souls let us love by all means, but not allow ourselves to be misled by beautiful bodies. This is one result of *śaucha*. It shows our own foulness as well as that of others; and inasmuch as it produces disgust of physical bodies, it indirectly helps the mind in the attainment of concentration. But it has also a direct bearing on the subject.

Our bodies are made up of three qualities—goodness, passion, and darkness. Health is the result when the quality of goodness (*satwa guna*) is predominant, and disease when darkness predominates. By *śaucha* the quality of goodness is made pure, it is freed from the two other qualities—*Raja* and *Tama* (passion and darkness); in other words,—and to use modern phraseology,— *śaucha* produces health. When there is health, there is cheerfulness and complacency. The unhealthy are generally moping and melancholy; but sound physical health engenders buoyancy and elasticity of spirit. When there is cheerfulness, it brings intentness, (*ekágratá*). It is the fixing of the mind to one train of ideas; but when the mind is not cheerful, it is impossible so to fix it. When there is *ekâgratâ*, and the mind is intent upon one subject, then there is *indriya jaya* (subjugation of senses). For all of us have seen that, when deeply engaged in one thought, we are not conscious of any external event, our senses are abstracted from the performance of their function, and we are said to be in abstraction. Where there is subjugation of the senses and perfect abstraction, the mind sees the soul. For what must one be cognizant of but his own soul, when one has made himself totally unconscious to the impressions conveyed by the senses? And seeing one's soul is Yoga. Thus we see how *śaucha*, through an unbroken chain of effects, leads to Yoga.

Next to purification, comes *santoṣa* (contentment). "The fruit of *santoṣa* is superlative felicity." Contentment is the fountain of true happiness. Our desires are infinite and insatiable, and lead but to sorrow. Happiness for which every one strives is not the result of enjoyment. There is a Persian saying, " Contentment makes one rich" nay, we say it makes one more than kings. A person is rich who has more than he desires, and, as one who is contented, has few desires—he is rich. We measure riches by wealth, but it is a false standard. The true measure of riches is our wants. If our wants be greater than our means to supply them, we are poor; but if our wants be few we are rich. Contentment is the true philosopher's stone. It diminishes our wants and multiplies our happiness. But we hear some to object that contentment is the bane of progress; the contented people are always stationary; that multiplication of our wants is a sign of civilization, and it is only among less advanced nations that we see the so-called virtue of contentment: civilized nations are ever progressive, never content. To all this we reply:—What is after all the result of all your vaunted civilization? Has it not made men heartless, greedy and selfish? Has it not sown discontent broad and wide? Does it not give rise to pains, envy and heart-burnings? Has it not turned all our energies to material improvements, external progress, and made us forget that we have a soul to save, immortality to achieve? Has materialistic philosophy made a single soul happy, or has it not cast a gloomy shroud of sadness and doubt over all our spiritual aspirations of futurity? No, this philosophy stands self-condemned, as it has failed to achieve its object, *viz.*, the increase of the sum total of human happiness. Nor do we admit that because a nation practises contentment it becomes incapable of progress and enterprise. Contentment only purges away the dross of self from our actions, and makes all our deeds shine with a lustre divine. It inspires the nation with love of justice and fair-play; and, since it takes away the petty, cold,-calculating greediness, which is the characteristic of most of the civilized nations, it makes us truly noble. Contentment is not a foe to progress, but it offers the necessary counterbalance to that spirit of insatiate hunger, which progress tends to generate.

Now we return to the fruit of *tapa* or taking trouble or exercise. "The prefection of the bodily senses by the removal of impurity is the fruit of austerity." It is a well-known law of nature that exercise strengthens our bodily organs; and that, if an organ is not properly exercised, it becomes imperfect. The system of *tapa* lays down minute rules for the perfection of the bodily senses. By a course of severe and rigorous discipline all our senses are sharpened and perfected. *Tapa* during these latter days of Indian history, has degenerated into physical penance and mortifications, totally unfruitful of the beneficial results contemplated. For a description of the various kinds of *tapas*, the reader is referred to treatises like Manu Sanhitâ, Yâjnyavalkya, &c. Any book on gymnastics will give more about the rules of *tapas* than we can do within the short space at our command. But, in passing, we may be allowed to remark that our *tapas* should not be confined to any one bodily organ, but to all. Thus, we should try to improve the keenness of our sight by looking steadily towards the stars, to make ourselves proof against heat and cold by bathing in cold water, during winter and so on. In fact, any practice tending towards the perfection of bodily senses is a *tapas*.

Fourthly, as to the fruits of incessant repetition of the word :—" Through *swadhyâya*, there is meeting with one's favorite deity." This requires no explanation. If we constantly and earnestly call upon a person, and if such a person does exist, it is but rational to suppose that he will answer our call. Deities or Devas are higher than *pitras* or spirits. Modern theology has named them angels, seraphs, cherubs, &c., while modern theosophy is pleased to call them elementals, spirits and elementaries. Some of these Devas are beneficient and others malignant ; however, both classess possess powerful attributes. In India, we have a class of religionists who are known as *devatâ-siddhas*, *i.e.*, those who have met with their special deity. Some worship Durgâ, others Ganeśâ, some Śiva, and so on. These persons, from intently repeating the name of a particular deity for a certain number of times, at last see that deity and receive certain powers as a reward of their labour. Some can cure peculiar diseases, others can find lost treasure, &c. That there is a good deal of imposition by them, and that all their vaunts and pretensions may not be true, is proved beyond doubt. But that there are genuine and real *devatâ-siddhas* is equally certain. But it is not a very high order of perfection after all, that we should aim at it. Rather we should leave the Devatâs to themselves, for they are potent to do evil as well as good, and it is not always easy to invoke them. Instead of worshipping any of these secondary deities, we should try to invoke none but the only one without a second, and devote to *Iswara pranidhâna*, the fruit of which is as follows :—

" Perfection in meditation (*samâdhi-siddhi*) comes from persevering devotion to the Lord." In fact, as we have said in the previous chapter, this path is the easiest, most simple, and pleasantest of all. " Love thy God with all thy heart, soul, and with all thy might," is the formula which explains the

CHAPTER VII.

adeptship of Lord Jesus and other saints. *Jnâna Yogis* are very few, but the *Bhakti Yoga*, being simple in theory and easy of practice, has been always popular with the masses. The essence of this system of Yoga is faith—faith in one's own-self, and faith in one's own God. But the path, though less difficult, is not all smooth sailing. While *Jnâna Yoga* is definite and certain of its results, the *Bhakti Yoga* is vague, indefinite and uncertain. Trance and ecstacy are the states which sometimes so fascinate the imagination of the *Bhakta*, that he thinks it the *ultima thule* of *samâdhi*, and does not wish to progress further. Moreover, there is more discordance of views among religionists than among philosophers. For, religion appeals more to the feelings than intuition, and consequently there is seldom found harmony among the saints of the world. No doubt both lead to the same goal, and it is a matter of choice, which of these one prefers.

CHAPTER VIII.
2.—Âsana.

The third aṅga of Yoga is âsana (posture). The best posture is that which is steady and pleasant. If we be uncomfortably seated, it is clear that our thoughts will be never collected. A good conscience, which follows from the practice of yama; and sound health which is the result of niyama, are no doubt very necessary. But given a clear conscience and sound health, the third requisite is good posture while practising Yoga. The later authors on Yoga mention some eighty-four different postures, e.g., Padmâsana, Yogâsana, Siddhâsana, Sukhâsana, and so on. But Patañjali is very wisely silent on this point, and leaves the question of âsana to be settled by everybody for himself. He only points out the conditions of a good âsana, and does not enter into details. As a guide for the beginner, we here quote some few of the postures.

The Viṣṇu Purâṇa gives the following directions :—" Sitting with the feet stretched out and so crossed as to touch the thighs, with the right hand stretched out and resting on the left, with the tongue fixed in the palate, and without bringing one row of teeth in contact with the other, with the eyes directed to the tip of the nose, and without glancing at any of the four quarters of the sky, let him meditate," &c.

The Buddhist method is :—" If the mode called pwankea be adopted, then the left leg is placed above the right and drawn close into the body, so that the toes of the left foot be placed evenly on the right thigh, and those of the right foot on the left thigh. But if the ts'inen-kea mode of sitting be preferred, then the right leg is to be put uppermost. The palm of the left hand should be placed in the hollow of the right, corresponding to the position of the legs. The next requirement is to straighten the body. Having first of all stretched the joints seven or eight times, let the spine be perfectly straight, neither curved nor humped, the head and neck upright, the nose exactly plumb with the navel, neither awry, nor slanting, nor up, nor down, but the whole face straight and perfectly fixed."

CHAPTER VIII.

According to the Persian method, the devotee sits on his hands, cross-legged, passing the outside of the right foot over the left thigh, and that of the foot over the right thigh; he then places his hands behind his back, and holds in his left hand the great toe of the right foot, and in the right hand the great toe of the left foot, fixing his eyes intently on the tip of the nose."

The aim of Yoga being to train the will-power, a steady posture should never be neglected. Determination and firmness of will appear as much from actions, as from the outward demeanour of the person. A strong-willed person will always sit upright, and walk with upraised head, straight and steadily; while a weak person will be always changing his posture, whether sitting or standing; his gait in motion is shambling, wavering and zigzag, and his every step betrays infirmity and want of resolution of the mind. Such a one can never sit at his ease for any length of time in one posture, but will be constantly shifting it. Therefore, it is of great importance to learn 'Âsana.' No doubt it will be found irksome to a degree in the beginning, to be sitting like a statue without motion, in one posture; but habit will make it pleasant.

The result or fruit of practising *âsana* is:—"There is no assault from the pairs," *i e.*, heat and cold, hunger and thirst, &c. By assuming a steady manly posture, our nerves are braced and tightened with the tightening of the body, and enable the body to resist heat and cold better, than a loose and weak one. Now for an example: if on a cold day you sit shivering and trembling and contorting yourself into diverse postures to feel warm, ten to one you will feel more cold; but if, on the contrary, you tight yourself up, erect your spine, and sit steadily in any one of the *âsanas* mentioned before, or in fact in any posture, you will at once feel a considerable diminution of cold and a pleasant increase of heat. The reason of this may be, that in sitting with our chest straight we inhale more oxygen, and our blood is more completely aerated than otherwise; and so enables us to keep up the normal temperature. In summer, when one is perspiring profusely and finds little relief from the fan, let him assume a good *âsana*, and witness with what a magic effect all the sweat vanishes and he feels comfortably cool. A steady *âsana* produces mental equilibrium, and thus explains some of the results which follow from its mastery. We can resist the claims of hunger and thirst for a long time, if we turn away our thoughts from them ; and *ásana*, (by diverting our minds from them and strengthening our will) produces the desired result.

The postures should be continued not only while practising Yoga, but always. While walking, let our steps fall firm and steady, and so in sleep, &c. We should regularly drill ourselves to perfection, and must never lose sight of these apparently trifling things.

CHAPTER IX.

4—Prâṇâyâma.

Prâyâṇâma is meant to restrain the inspiration and expiration. Prâna is synonymous with breath and life. It has both these meanings. The ancient philosophers of India had, at a very early period of their investigations, discovered the grand truth that life, as found in higher animals, is dependent upon oxygen. Modern science but confirms their view. Of the " tripod of life," composed of the lungs, heart, and brain, the latter two are ordinarily beyond the control of our direct volition. The heart will beat, and the hemispheres of the cerebrum will go on with their work giving birth to thought, &c., (as a rule) independent of will. These two hemispheres, as well as the heart, are not under our control. The muscular fibres of the heart contract and dilate from the action or direct influence of the brain as well as the nervous ganglia centred in its very substance. The action of the heart, on the whole, is involuntary ; though sometimes, as under the influence of great fear or excitement, its motion may be accelerated or retarded considerably beyond normal limits. Unconscious cerebration goes on simultaneously with the impulse of the heart, and then manifested as conscious ideas, independent of the will. The heart is the principal organ which, by propelling the blood through the lungs aerates and purifies it, and, by distributing it through the arteries, keeps up the animal life. To suspend animal life, therefore, we must suspend the action of the heart, so that the various organs, such as the eye, the ear, &c., may become for the time paralysed, and the spirit liberated. All the senses work harmoniously so long as they receive a pure blood supply from the heart ; and when that is stopped or vitiated their action also stops or becomes dull or deadened. But as the action of the heart has been shown to be involuntary, to influence it we must act through the lungs,—in other words, through the breath. Prâṇâyâma (or regulation of the breath) treats, consequently, of all those methods which temporarily suspend the functions of animal life, and thereby facilitate the liberation of the spirit. There are different modes of bringing about this result, but the one proposed by the Yogi through the regulation of the breath, is the easiest, and safest, and, what is its greatest recommendation, it requires no external accessories. Fumigation, dancing, music, &c., have been employed by various mystics to bring about trance, but all these mean the help of external adjuncts. The Aryan mind, panting after absolute liberty, would never be indebted to anything beyond its own soul. It always strove to find all its resources within itself, and thus it became really, and, in the true sense of the word, free. Music and fumigating pastilles or essences and spirits, balsams and ointments, may not always be with you, and if by Prâṇâyâma you can bring about the same result as the Magi by his incense, or the wizard by his ointment, or the *Faqir* by his music, where then is the necessity of all these appliances? They seem to a true Yogi as so many fetters and hindrances, rather than helps. Thus the extreme simplicity of the methods employed by our forefathers strikes us at every turn, and gives ample proof of their wisdom and knowledge of psychology.

To understand fully the action of respiration on life, some knowledge of physiology is absolutely necessary. With this purpose we give below a short account of the three organs—the heart, lungs and brain—and shall try to show their relation with each other and action and inter-action.

To begin with the heart:—It is a small muscular sac of the size of the human fist inclined to the left side of the chest, underneath the ribs. Its apex corresponds with the left nipple and is broad at the base, resembling in form a betel leaf. Its colour is dark purple. The inside of the sack is divided into two chambers, by a muscular wall running mid-way, and called the right and left divisions. The impure blood, which is of a dark color, comes, through the various veins of the body, into one principal vein, which discharges its contents into the right half of the heart. From the right chamber, the impure blood goes to the lungs, where, being purified by absorbing oxygen, it comes to the left side of the heart, and is thence driven to the whole body by the arterial system. The two chambers of the heart contain different kinds of blood—the right half containing the dark, purple, venous blood; and the left, bright, crimson, arterial blood. The effect of the dark venous blood on the nerves is to deaden their susceptibility, while that of the bright arterial blood is to quicken the vitality; the venous blood produces asphyxia, because it contains a good deal of carbonic acid, the product of muscular waste; while the arterial blood sustains life, because it contains a great

CHAPTER IX. 39

proportion of oxygen. In the economy of the human system, the heart serves as a general caterer, which supplies nourishment to the whole body.

The lungs are intimately related to the heart. They are two large organs situated in the thoracic cavity containing air-cells. Under a microscope a small section of the substance of the lungs, if examined, will be found to consist of infinite minute cavities, lined with a very thin membrane. The blood remains outside of these cavities, which are full of air. The exchange of the carbonic acid of the blood with the oxygen of the air does not take place direct, but through the intervention of this thin membrane.

The brain is the organ of the mind, the seat of intellect and ideas. The centre whence the nerve-force for the production of combined respiratory movement appears to issue, is situated in the interior of that part of medulla oblongata, from which the pneumogastric nerves arise. This part of the medulla oblongata is the nerve centre, which gives rise to the respiratory movements and through which impulses conveyed from distant parts are reflected. With every beating of the heart and the heaving of the breath, the brain cerebrates. The effect of breathing on thought is very well explained by Swedenborg, which we quote below:—"Thought commences and corresponds with respiration. The reader has before attended to the presence of the heaving over the body; now let him *feel* his *thoughts*, and he will see that they too heave with the mass. When he entertains a long thought, he draws a long breath; when he thinks quickly, his breath vibrates with rapid alternation; when the tempest of anger shakes his mind, his breath is tumultuous; when his soul is deep and tranquil, so is his respiration; when success inflates him, his lungs are as timid as his concepts. Let him make trial of the contrary; let him endeavour to think in long stretches, at the same time that he breathes in fits, and he will find that it is impossible; that in this case, the chopping will needs mince his thoughts. Now, this mind dwells in the brain, and it is the brain, therefore, which shares the varying fortunes of the breathing. Inward thoughts have inward breaths, and purer spiritual breaths hardly mixed with material."

We have said before that *prâṇâyâma* aims at suspending the functions of the physical and mental bodies, and that it tries to do so, among other things, by reducing the beating of the heart through restraining the breath. This is the highest aim of *prâṇâyâma*.

But now-a-days those who practise Yoga and *prânâyâma* generally do not think of reducing the normal action of the heart. They wish to harmonise the faculties by slow, steady and synchronous breathing. The mind may be compared to a gas flame, which is being constantly agitated by the uneven flow of the gas from the pipe, and not being well protected by properly constructed chimneys and shades from external air; the blood which the heart sends to the brain is the gas which sustains the flame of the mind; and owing to the various passions and feelings, the supply of blood to the brain is not always constant; and the mind flickers and flutters, and sheds but a tremulous light. Therefore, by the practice of the *prânâyâmic* method, the Yogi, consciously or unconsciously, sends a constant, uninterrupted and equable stream of blood to the brain, and tries to keep the flame ever steady.

The methods of *prânâyâma* are infinite, and a vast majority of them very difficult to practise. Among the Persians, it is known by the name of *habs-i-dam*, confining of breath. The technical name of inspiration is *puraka*; expiration is called *rechaka*, and restraining of breath is known as *kumbhaka*. One of the methods in general practice is the following:—Close with the thumb of the right hand the right nostril, and breathe slowly through the left one, repeating seven times the word Om; then close both the nostrils and restrain the breath for a space of time sufficient for repeating the sacred formula *Om tat sat* (or any other favourite *mantra*) fourteen times; and then breathe out through the right nostril, repeating the mystic syllable seven times. This should be practised continually till the Yogi can sit in *kumbhaka* for minutes together. It can be done by slowly increasing the period of *kumbhaka* by increasing the duration from fourteen to twenty-one times, and so on by every increment of seven. There are ordinary *grihastas* even, who have carried the practice of *kumbhaka* to such lengths that they can easily restrain their breath for five or six minutes. A beginner needs not despair if he can, after the practice of a month, withhold his breath for a minute,—as a minute will seem like an hour.

Another method peculiar to the Persian is the following:— Sitting in a good *âsana*, inspire slowly, repeating the word *nêst* till the lungs are so much filled that the pressure of the diaphragm is felt at the navel; then incline the head towards the right breast,

CHAPTER IX. 41

reciting the word *hasti*, and expel the breath; and raise the head up, take a deep inspiration, repeating the word *magar*; afterwards uttering *yâzdâñ*, and, inclining the head on the left side, expel the breath. "The devotee makes no pause between the words thus recited." The formula is *nêst hasti, magar yâzdâñ.* "There is no existence save God." In this system, there is no *kumbhaka*, but *rechaka* and *puraka* only, and the period between them is gradually lessened, so that in one minute the devotee repeats the formula more than a hundred times. We saw a Muhammadan friend of ours practising this method; but he had substituted, instead of the above words, the formula *Allah Hu,*--raising his head with *Allah* and throwing it down with *Hu.* He repeated them so very quickly, and threw his head from one side to the other so incessantly, that within a short time he felt exhausted, and afterwards informed us that he could go into a trance within five minutes by continuing it. Another modification of the same method is that in which the devotee raises and drops his head and utters several formulæ in one breath, gradually increasing their number. This latter method is more calm and less exciting, and the duration of *kumbhaka*, being continually increased, approaches more to the Hindu system, and is the real *habs-i-dam,*--restraining of the breath.

Another Persian method is:—"The worshipper, having closed the right nostril, enumerates the names of God from one to sixteen times, and, whilst counting, draws his breath upwards, after which he repeats it twenty-two times lets the breath escape out of the right nostril, and, whilst counting, propels the breath aloft, thus passing from the six *khans* or stages to the seventh; until, from the intensity of imagination, he arrives at a state in which he thinks that his soul and breath are bound like the jet of a fountain to the crown of the head." After this, there follows a very peculiar and mystical passage:—"As causing the breath to mount to the crown of the head is a power peculiar to the most eminent persons, so whoever can convey his breath and soul together to that part becomes the viceregent of God." We do not say that we have fully understood the above passage, but having some knowledge of the symbolical writing of our forefathers, we think that the above sentence should be construed not in its literal sense, but occult signification. Breath is the vehicle of thought, soul or *jivâtmâ*; this *jivâtmâ* must be purified and united with the *paramâtmâ*, whose seat is represented to be the crown of the head. When this unification is complete, man becomes one with Brahma.

The seven stages alluded to above are the following:—(1) between the organ of generation and anus; (2) the root of the organ; (3) the navel; (4) the heart; (5) the throat, (6) between the eyebrows; and (7) the crown of the head. The first is the seat of the earth; the second, of the water; the third, of the fire; the fourth, of air; the fifth, of the ether; the sixth, of the mind; and the seventh, of the Paramâtma. The human soul must pass through all these stages before it can join with its original source. The first is the cause of the physical body, the second, of vital force, the third, of the astral body or *Liṅga Sarîra*, the fourth, of the aerial body or *Kâmrûpa*, the fifth, of the etherial body or elemental spirit, the sixth is the human soul, and the seventh needs no explanation. A Yogí, as long as he does not conquer the first step, stands in need of solid food; when he reaches the second stage, he can dispense with it, and would require only liquid food; and the more he progresses, the more subtle becomes his nourishment. We have rather digressed from our subject intentionally, in order to warn the unguided reader of Yoga not to take literally whatever he finds in those ancient occult books. Nay, he may meet with some misled and misleading Yogis who will seriously tell him to practise *prâṇâyâma* by drawing his breath forcibly up to the Brahmarandhra,—a feat which, under the present constitution of our body, is simply impossible. Ignorant, self-taught Yogis are always exposed to the danger of degenerating into Haṭha Yoga. We know of a lady who, putting a wrong interpretation on a passage in the Bhagavat Gitâ, practised *prâṇâyâma* all night and became mad; and it was after many days that she regained her intellect, after being daily mesmerised by her brother.

Buddhists enumerate four kinds of respiration:—"1st, the windy; 2nd, gasping; 3rd, emotional; and 4th, pure respiration. The first three modes are unharmonised; the last is harmonised. When the breath passing in and out of the nostrils is perceived by the noise it makes, it is called windy; second, although there is no noise in breathing, yet, when the respiration is broken and uneven, as though it comes not through a clear passage, it is gasping; the third is emotional, when, although there is no noise or gasping, still the respiration is not equable or smooth. Proper and pure respiration is that in which there is neither noise nor gasping nor

CHPTER IX. 43

uneven breathing, but it is calm and regular, the sign of an equable and well balanced mind."

Another method of regulating the breath is as follows :— Close with the thumb of your right hand, the right ear, and with that of the left hand, the left ear. Close with the two index fingers the two eyes, place the two middle fingers upon the two nostrils, and let the remaining fingers press upon the upper and the lower lips. Draw a deep breath, close both the upper nostrils at once, and swallow the breath. This act of swallowing, if well done, will make a partial vacuum in the passages of the nostrils and the mouth, and there will be felt a strain upon the auditory nerves which will be partially paralysed, followed by confused humming in the ears Keep the breath inside as long as you conveneintly can ; then expire it slowly, and so on. Swallowing of the breath not only facilitates the deadening of the nerves of the ear, but after some time the eye in its turn will be affected. Strange coruscations similarly, blue and white flashes like the lightning, will pass before the eyes. These lights must not be mistaken for the pure astral light of which we will speak soon, but they owe their existence to the physical pressure which falls upon the optic nerve."

"Another mode, which is rather dangerous, is by directing the current of the breath towards the heart. Breath is drawn in such a way that the left lung is distended more than the right, and presses upon the heart. But the process being somewhat perilous, and the present writer having pledged his word to his instructor not to reveal it without his express permission, though there is after all nothing much in it worth keeping back, he forbears for the present from entering into details. Broad hints, however, have been given in the foregoing lines, which, if understood and practised, might lead to speedy attainment of perfection in *prâṇâyâma* than any other method."

Sanskrit authors of comparatively modern period unnecessarily complicate this simple system of *prâṇâyâma*, as taught by the original teacher, Patañjali, by enumerating five different kinds of *vâyus* or winds. These *vâyus* preside over the various functions in the human economy, and are called--1st, the Prâṇâ vâyu, or the ascending air with its seat at the fore end or tip of the nose ; 2nd, the Apâna vâyu or the descending air with its seat in the anus ; 3rd, the Vyâna vâyu moves in all directions, and is present in all parts of the body ; 4th, the Udâna vâyu is the ascending air, situated in the throat; 5th, Samâna vâyu, the air inside the body, which helps the digestion of food. "These five vital airs originate in the active attribute of ether and other elements. With the five organs action they constitute what is designated "the life-sac." From the above classification of *vâgus* and their intimate connection with the life-sac or *anna-maya koṣa* it has been argued that to suspend, though temporarily, the active phenomena of life one must have control over these five winds. But to us all this seems to be altogether unnecessary. Proper regulation of the Prâṇavâyu is sufficient for the purpose, and we need not try to learn the method of regulating the other winds.

Prânâyama is both natural as well as artificial. Whenever a person thinks intensely on a subject, his breath of itself assumes proper prânâyamic motion. Observe the respiration of one in deep sleep and you will get some idea of what should be the proper duration, etc., of the breath for a Yogi. A Yogi but consciously produces that state of respiration which is favourable for contemplation, as others produce occasionally and unconsciously. Often one can in the stillness of night, when sleep does not visit his eyelids, and ideas flow uncalled and unasked for put himself to sleep by merely drawing in and expelling breath simultaneously and synchronously with that of any other person sleeping near him. Thus often by bringing one's breath in harmony with that of another he can enjoy the same state of felicity as the other; and though we cannot vouch for the truth of the theory from our own personal experience, yet we say there might be something in that saying, which asserts: "bring thy breath in harmony with that of another, and thou wilt know what passes in his mind."

The hygienic effect of prânâyama is beyond doubt. We have seen a friend curing small ailments like headache or approach of fever and cold, by simply practising prânâyama.

There are many points in connection with regulation of breath which we now-a-days class among superstitions, since we have lost the rationale. Thus it is said that one's undertakings will all prove successful if he commences it when he respires through his right nostril. Similarly, if you start from your home to visit a friend, and wish to know whether you will find him or not at home, examine your breath; if it flows through the right nostril, you will see him, otherwise not. There are others who could tell the hour of the day from the motion of their breath.

CHAPTER IX.

It is said, that in every healthy person the breath (technically known as *sura*) changes from one nostril to the other at well-established regular intervals, and thus from its being right or left-sided, those practised in it can approximately say the hour of the day.

Now, for the fruit or result of prâṇâyâma:—"Thereby is removed the obscuration of the light." The light here alluded to is the pure *sâttvik* light which the Yogi sees in his heart when in deep contemplation. It may be the same light which the mesmerised subjects of Baron Reichenbach saw issuing from the poles of the magnet, &c. When mesmerising, we have invariably found that the first thing which the mesmerised person sees, as soon as his eyes are closed in utter darkness, as black as night. Slowly, in this darkness there are seen flashes of blue light which growing stronger, the subject begins to see a blue atmosphere surrounding him. This is the *chiṭṭâkâsâ* of the Vedântins, the region of imagination. Pictures and persons seen in this light are generally the products of the brain of the sensitive, and have no objective reality. This light gives way to pure white electric light, very brilliant, and described as more pleasant, clear and luminous than that of the sun. This is the *chidâkâsâ* proper, the light of intelligence or soul, through which the clairvoyant sees.

A further result of prâṇâyâma is "that the mind becomes fit for acts of attention." This requires no explanation. When there is harmony in breathing, there also ensues harmony in ideas, and the mind becomes better adapted to acts of attention.

NOTE.

The importance of *Prânâyâma* is recognized by some of the celebrated medical authorities of the present day as may be gathered from the following extract from " A Lecture on means for the Prolongation of Life " delivered by Sir Hermann Weber, M D., F.R. C.P., before the Royal College of Physicians of London and published is the *British Medical Journal* for December 5th, 1903. It in needless to add that " Respiratory Exercises " mean *Prânâyâma*.

RESPIRATORY EXERCISES.

"The remarkable improvement in the heart's nutrition and action is, I think, to a great degree caused by the deep inspirations which are necessitated by the act of climbing, especially steady and prolonged climbing. This consideration has led me to pay particular attention to respiratory exercises, which since then have been very useful to myself and many others, especially persons with weak heart muscles. I make no claim of originality for these exercises; they are only a modification of several older systems of gymnastics. As in walking and other bodily exercises, the amount and modus of respiratory movements which are useful, greatly vary with the inidividual condition, and must be adapted to the latter. It is often injurious in cases of weakness of the heart or lungs, or the sequelæ of pneumonia or pleurisy or other acute disease, especially influenza, to begin at once with forced respiratory movements. I have mostly commenced with moderately deep inspirations and expirations, continued during three to five minutes, once or twice a day, and have gradually increased the exercise to ten minutes or a quarter of an hour. The depth of each inspiration and expiration, is likewise to be only gradually increased. At the beginning, a sixth or a quarter or half a minute, for every inspiration and every expiration ought to be sufficient; if this is well borne, each act may be gradually prolonged in duration, so that in the majority of cases each inspiration and each expiration may be brought up to a minute. All the movements are to be made slowly, not rapidly. I usually advise to inspire in the erect position, with raised arms and closed mouth, and to bend down the body during expiration, so that the fingers touch the ground or the toes. By degrees one can learn to make several up-and-down movements during every inspiration, and bend and raise the body several times during the expiration. By this alternate bending and raising of the body we gain the additional advantage of strengthening the lumbar muscles and, through this, successfully combating the tendency to lumbago. Another useful combination with the respiratory exercises is the turning of the body round the axis of the spinal column, alternately with deep inspiration from left to right, and with expiration from right to left, with half raised arms. By this movement we bring into action some of the muscles of the spine which are apt to be only imperfectly used by most persons in advanced years; and the stiffness of the neck and spine, and the tendency to stoop, so common in old people, can be to some degree corrected by this kind of movement, if commenced early enough and practised regularly and thoroughly. The swinging of the arms round the shoulder-joint is, likewise, a useful combination. * * * In addition to the influence on the circulation, the respiratory movements keep up the nutrition and efficiency of the lungs themselves, which undergo in old age a kind of atrophy; the walls of the smallest divisions and air-cells become thinner, and a kind of senile emphysema in these exercises is to some degree prevented. Another important influence consists in maintaining the elasticity of the chest walls, which are apt to become stiff in old age, and thus to interfere with free movements of the lungs and the pleura.

" If for some reason the erect position should be inconvenient, the mere respiratory movements can be made also in the horizontal and sitting positions. I have already alluded to the additional advantage of the compression of the abdomen and the blood vessels and organs contained in the abdominal cavity, and we may further point out that the action of the serous membranes, of the pleura, the pericardium, and the peritoneum are also beneficially influenced by the deep respiratory movements; they constitute a kind of massage to the lungs, the thoracic walls, pericardium, and heart (Sir Lauder Brunton). * * *

" We must, however, not be satisfied with the few minutes of respiratory exercises, but we must make a habit of taking at several other times of each day deep inspirations and expirations, especially while walking. Breathing exercises are especially useful to literary workers, statesmen, professional men, and others who are unable to take one of the usual modes of exercise. The most convenient time for practising them is in the morning before or after the bath, when the body is loosely covered with flannel. I ought to add that they are not suitable for very delicate persons; they are, for instance, injurious in great dilatation of the heart with or without valvular disease. * * * * On the other hand, their judicious use may be regarded as one of the preventives of diseases of the lungs, and can also be rendered beneficial in the later stages of convalescence from acute disease, and under medical guidance in some apyretic forms of chronic tuberculosis."

CHAPTER X.

5.—*Pratyâhâra*.

"Pratyâhâra is as it were the accommodation of the senses to the nature of the mind in the absence of concernment with each one's own object. This fruit of this is the complete subjection of the senses." Mind in ordinary men is the slave of the senses. If our sensations are pleasant, we feel pleasure; if painful, we are pained. Senses not only domineer, but tyrannize over the mind. Therefore, when the Yogi has passed through all the four stages enumerated above, *i.e.*, *yama, niyama, âsana and prânâyâma*, he should try to accommodate his senses to the nature of his mind. When he does not wish to see, let not external things make any impression on his retina, though he may have his eyes wide open. When he has no mind to hear, let no external sound make any impression on the nerves of the cochlea, and so on; not only he should be the negative master over his senses, *i.e.*, restraining them from their functions whenever he wishes, but he should be so complete and perfect master over them, that they should respond like obedient servants to every call of his mind. When his mind thinks of a pleasant picture, let the nerves of the eye catch up the thought and *show* it to him in objective reality. When he *thinks* of a sound, let the ears responding to the thought make him *hear* it as well. When he imagines of a smell, let his olfactory nerves *feel* the sensation. In fact, *pratyâhâra* is that state in which the subjective world overcomes the objective, and imagination is exalted to such a pitch that all its pictures stand forth vividly on the canvas of objectivity. The practice of prânâyâma as invariably induces the pratyâhâra as the passes of a strong mesmeriser produce sleep. Yoga has been very happily termed self-mesmerisation, in which the subject is the mystic's own body. As in mesmerism, the operator can make his subject see any sight, hear any sound, smell any odour, taste any taste, or feel any sensation which the operator *imagines*, so the Yogi, who has reached the fifth stage, has a similar control over the organs of his body. He asserts the supremacy of the mind over the body by the same will-force as the ordinary mesmeriser, and as the latter makes his patient unconscious to all external sensations, so that a gun may be fired without his hearing it;

pungent odours like that of ammonia may be held near the nose without his smelling it; brilliant light may pass unnoticed when focussed on his eyes, for the *iris* remains inert; pungent chillies may be placed on the tongue, and he will swallow them without showing any sign of pain; so does many a Yogi get supremacy over his own body so as to defy sensation. Pratyâhâra is not a distinct method in itself, but is a result of prâṇâyâma. There are no rules laid down for the subjugation of the senses, as there are for the regulation of the breath; but it comes in the wake of the other four processes. When in practising prâṇâyâma the *âbharana* or obscuration of light is removed and the Yogi sees the pellucid Chidâkâsha (the pure spiritual light), he enjoys such pleasant sensations that of itself his mind is transferred from taking cognition of the external things to internal ideas, and the senses become inactive.

Thus we have treated of the five externalities of Yoga—the Bahiranga, as they are called. The *mind* has not yet been reached, as up to this time we have been dealing only with the *body*. The last of these five stages culminates in the suppression of the senses and total subjugation of the body to the mind. The remaining three stages treat of the methods of subjecting the *mind* to the *soul*, and these processes are called *antaranga* (internal) in relation to the *body*; while considered in relation to the *soul* they are Bahiranga.

TABLE OF METHODS.

I		II		III
Methods culminating in the subjugation of the body.		Methods culminating in the subjugating of the *mind*.		Method of union of the human Âtma with the Paramâtma.
1. Yama ... 2. Niyama ... 3. Âsana ... 4. Prâṇâyâma 5. Pratyâhâra	Bahiranga to the 2nd class.	6. Dhyâna ... 7. Dhâraṇa 8. Savikalpa-Samâdhi	Antaranga in relation to class I, but Bahiranga to class III.	Nirvikalpa Samâdhi.

CHAPTER XI.

(Pratyâhâra and Anæsthetics.)

We have said before, that there are other methods of suspending the nerves of consciousness, or physical life, besides Prâṇâyâma and Pratyâhâra. Some of them are occult; in short, the agency through which these results are produced is not properly understood by modern scientists; there are others which may be termed scientific in the limited acceptation of the term. All these methods tend to produce unconsciousness, to suspend vitality, and to bring on temporary death. A man in this state of Pratyâhâra, whether induced by medicinal drugs, or by the occult manipulation of *vâyû* and *âkâs* is little removed from a vegetable in the external manifestations of life; but his mental consciousness is at the same time much intensified.

The medicinal drugs which produce Pratyâhâra are known as anæsthetics. ".When inhaled in the form of vapour, they possess the property of destroying consciousness (?) and at the same time causing insensibility to pain." The most important of them are (1) chloroform, (2) ether, (3) nitrous oxide gas, etc. Ether was formerly in greater demand than at present; now chloroform reigns supreme; while nitrous oxide gas, also known as the laughing gas, is used for smaller operations, by Dentists. The principal condition of their administration is the same, as that required in Yoga, *viz.*,— "the patient should fast for 5 or 6 hours before chloroform is exhibited," so also " before administering the nitrous oxide gas ; the only precaution to be observed is that a meal should not have been recently taken." Messrs. Lallemand, Perin and Duroy observe :—" We have usually experimented [with chloroform] only on fasting animals, but once we happened to give chloroform to a dog, whilst it was digesting a full meal. The course of the phenomena was so irregular and so grave (the animal dying a short time afterwards) that we considered it our duty to record the experiment. In all experiments wherein the dogs were fasting, the mark of etherism was regular." But in submitting to " inhalation three dogs, a short time after they had taken food, the results were incomplete. The animals betrayed a painful anxiety, and rejected the food which loaded the stomach, the vomiting relieved them."

The nitrous oxide gas is the safest as an anæsthetic, leaving no injurious results. It doest not act chemically on the blood, and is soon eliminated out of the system when natural respiration is commenced. The action of chloroform in its various stages towards anæsthesia will do for an illustration :—

"When inhaled in small doses, it produces a slight species of inebriation, with some impairment of vision and common sensibility, consciousness remaining. The sensation produced by these small doses are usually of a pleasurable character." In the second stage, "if the inhalation be continued longer, the patient passes into a dreamy (?) state, sometimes with considerable mental excitement, but with loss of common sensibility." This stage corresponds with Pratyâhâra, when the Yogi loses common physical sensibility, but still retains consciousness. By carrying on the inhalation "the patient loses the power of voluntary motion, and he passes into unconsciousness ; then there is an inclination of the eyes upwards, and complete suspension of the mental faculties." This in Yoga corresponds to *savikalpa samâdhi*. Here modern medical science stops, and does not profess to go beyond. It has studied with great care and precaution, taken note of the minute changes which the *body* of the patient undergoes successively, but has not been equally successful in tracing the mental side of the picture. The science of Yoga steps in to supply the hiatus. If its results are to be credited (and we do not see why they should not), then we must perforce differ from the scientists who would have us believe that the last stage of anæsthesia is loss of consciousness. We are taught by those who have *experimented* with the *mind*, that the last stage, far from being loss of consciousness, is the highest and absolute state of consciousness which the human spirit, in its present stage of development, is capable of. Loss of memory which *ordinary* men experience when returning to their normal condition from a state of anæsthesia is no more proof of loss of consciousness than the *Sushuptiavasthâ* (the state of profound dreamless sleep). It requires special training to transfer the spiritual consciousness back into the physical consciousness. Some are naturally endowed with this faculty, and are born seers and magicians ; while others can develope it by a painful and laborious course of mental training, and are known as Adepts, Yogis, &c.

CHAPTER XI.

Some of the results of anæsthesia and the conditions of its administration throw a curious side-light on the truth of Yoga and the phenomena observed in Pratyâhâra. We give the following in confirmation of our assertion from a book on Chloroform by Dr. A. E. Samson, M. B. In the second stage " the senses become affected, frequently, the sounds in the room are exaggerated in their intensity, the tickling of the clock becomes like the falling of a ponderous hammer. The surrounding objects become dim and as it were dissolve in light, and then a veil enwraps them all. A strange effect is the phenomena of narcotic reminiscence. Events of the past life may be recalled, conversations may be repeated, and actions reproduced. I have heard a young girl, throughout the whole course of a surgical operation, sing, ' Beautiful star ' correctly, word for word and note for note." Similarly the precautions, necessary in the administration of anæsthetics, are almost the same as required by the Yogi Thus, to quote the same authority : —" Of all conditions of system, probably the worst to bear chloroform is *alcoholism*. It is a most note-worthy fact that when we look over the records of death from chloroform, we find that very many have occurred in *hard drinkers*. Intemperance induces a state of system most inimical to chloroform." For chloroform substitute **Yoga**, and it will be equally true. " The average age at which death from chloroform has occurred is 30, *the married are almost twice the number*." Here again we see the necessity of celibacy and the early practice of Yoga.

CHAPTER XII.

Antaranga Yoga.

The Psychic or super-normal powers, as enumerated by Patañjali, are many. Men can acquire them by certain training, a training which requires the development of spiritual faculties dormant in every man. That training has been divided into two parts :—Bahiranga (External or Subsidiary) and Antaranga (Internal or Primary). The Bahiranga consist of five parts, viz., Yama, Niyama Âsana, Prâṇâyâma, Pratyâhâra. Yama enjoins the observance of the following five rules :—1, Not to injure any living being (Ahinsâ); 2, Never to tell a lie and always to speak the truth, (Satya); 3, Never to steal another's property (Asteya); 4, Always to be pure and chaste, or celibacy (Brahmacharya); 5, Never to covet any thing (Aparigraha).

The Niyama enjoins the observance of the following :—
1. Be always pure, and observe the rules of purification. (For a detailed account of these, see "Daily Practice of the Hindus," recently published);
2. Be always content;
3. Observe austerity and asceticism ;
4. Study sacred books ;
5. Be perseveringly devoted to God.

The rules of Âsana or the postures are various. There are some 84 postures in which a Yogi can sit, some six of which are more important.

The rules of Prâṇâyâma or regulation of breath have already been given before.

Lastly, Pratyâhâra is the accommodation of the senses to the nature of the mind, or, in other words, the complete subjection of the senses.

The above are then the externalities of Yoga on which we need not dwell longer. They may be summed up in the following thirteen rules :—
1. Do not injure any living creature, but love all.
2. Always speak the truth.
3. Never commit theft (or wrongly take another's property).
4. Observe chastity and celibacy.
5. Forsake covetousness.
6. Be always pure in body and mind.

CHAPTER XII.   55

7. Be always contented.
8. Observe austerities and learn endurance.
9. Study sacred books and repeat sacred formulas.
10. Love the Lord with all thy heart and soul.
11. While practising Yoga, sit in a posture which is comfortable and easy.
12. Being so seated, regulate your breath by observing the rules of inspiring, expiring and retaining of breath.
13. Completely subdue all your senses and bring them in harmony with mind.

The observance of the above thirteen rules will prepare the aspirant for the attainment of higher powers. How to attain them is the immediate object of our discussion. All psychic powers are obtained and wonders worked through sanyama. This sanyama is the harmonious and simultaneous working of the three faculties or conditions of mind, called Dhâranâ, Dhyâna, and Samâdhi. These three constitute the internal or the primary or the essential part of Yoga. . We shall now enter upon a detailed description of these.

Dhâranâ is the fixing of the thinking principle (chitta) to a particular locality. This is the definition of Patañjali, and requires explanation to make its meaning clear. When the mind is bound up in a particular object or thinks only of a particular thing, it is said to hold (dhâranâ) that thing. The *effort* to catch hold of the object, and to keep it before the mind's eye, or, in other words, the *effort* to keep the mind fixed on a particular object, is dhârana. In Yoga, mind is fixed consecutively on various parts of the body, for example, on the navel, on the heart, on the throat. &c. A little experience will show that it is a difficult task to bind up the *chitta* or mind within a specified locality. Try to concentrate your mind, for example, on your heart, and try to keep it within the limit prescribed, and you will find it will soon slide out of it, roving about everywhere else, rather be confined to the place where you would like to have it. Or, to take another example, try to imagine and realise the picture of a flower, say rose. The *effort* in catching hold of the idea of the rose and keeping it before the mental eye is what is meant by the word Dhâranâ, as used by Patañjali Or, to take another example from the Hindu system of worship. A man is a worshipper of Śiva, when he enters on the path of mentally worshipping Śiva, sits in an easy posture, puts down the physical agitation by regulating his breath, composes his mind, and then practises *dhâranâs*; *i.e.*, he closes his eyes, and makes mental effort to picture the figure of Śiva. When this effort succeeds, the picture is developed and comes out prominently and distinctly in the field of mental vision. Here is then the consummation of the dhâranâ of the devotee.

After dhâranâ comes *dhyâna*, which is defined to be the course of uniform modification of knowledge in that place where the internal organ (chitta) is fixed in Dhâranâ. The word Dhyâna has been translated in English by the word contemplation. In contemplation, as above defined there is a uniform course of knowledge of the object of Dhâranâ. That is to say, in contemplation the mind performs two operations, it uniformly is conscious of the object of Dhâranâ; and it rejects every other thought incongruous with the above. The difference between the Dhâranâ and the Dhyâna consists in this: the first is the fixing of attention on a particular object or thought, out of many; but it supposes that there are other thoughts also in the mental field, along with the idea on which attention is directed. But in contemplation, all such extraneous thoughts are rejected and driven out, and the mind is fixed on the particular thought which reigns supreme and excludes all other thoughts; and the mind is conscious and cognisant of that idea and of no other, and does not allow any other idea to distract its attention.

After dhâranâ and dhyâna, comes Samâdhi. In contemplation or dhyâna the consciousness, uniform and without break, flows in one channel, *i.e.*, of the object of contemplation. In Samâdhi, this state of mental concentration reaches its culmination. It is defined to be the same contemplation or Dhyâna, when it arises only about a substance or object of sense, and is then like nonexistence of itself. When by constant practice of contemplation, the consciousness of all other objects than the object contemplated is completely lost, and when the mind is intent upon that contemplated object only, that oneness of mind is Samâdhi.

The three states—dhâranâ, dhyâna and samâdhi—rise by gradual gradations. In dhâranâ there is an *effort* to fix the mind on the object to be contemplated; in Dhyâna that object having risen vividly before the mental vision, there is an effort to *concentrate* the consciousness in that object, to the exclusion of every other idea; in samâdhi, this effort having succeeded, the mind loses, as if its own form, and becomes one with the object contem-

CHAPTER XII.

plated. These three—dhâranâ, dhyâna and samâdhi—will thus be apparent to be but the various stages of one mental effort or work, viz., the effort of concentration. There is no difference in kind between them, but only one of degree. These three conjointly are called Sanyama. Every effort of concentration consists of these three parts. What is then the result of Sanyama. The result is the attainment of

The first psychic power.

The light of Prajnâ or soul bursts forth when one has mastered or has obtained full control over Sanyama. When by constant practice and training one can perform sanyama about any object with ease and for long, the light of spiritual intelligence then manifests itself Through and by the medium of that light, knowledge of higher or sukṣma universe is obtained. Through that astral light wonders are wrought, and the so-called miracles performed.

APPENDIX I.
A BRIEF SKETCH OF VEDANTA AND YOGA.

Q.—Who is the *adhikâri*, or the person qualified to learn Vedanta and Yoga?

A.—He who is pure in his thoughts, mild in his words, and being free from all evil deeds, is benevolent towards all; who performs all the duties prescribed by the Śástras and Vedas; who moving in this world is not ensnared by it, and who has a burning, longing, panting and yearning after emancipation.

Q.—How should such a *mumukṣu* acquire self-knowledge?

A.—By means of the four *sádhanas* :—

(1). Distinguishing between the real and the non-real, the phenomena and the noumena, the eternal and the transient, realising that Brahma is the only truth.

(2). Performing works from the most disinterested motives, doing good for the sake of good, without expecting any reward here or hereafter.

(3). Having faith, endurance, self-control, passivity, abstinence, and intensity of thought.

(4). A strong desire for Nirvána.

Q.—What is the subject of Vedanta?

A.—To prove that the Paramâtmâ and Jivâtmâ are one and the same in essence—the human spirit being the reflection of the Divine Spirit.

Q.—What is the necessity of such a knowledge?

A.—The aim of all systems of philosophy is to acquire freedom from pain. Worldly philosophies, like medicine, etc., give momentary relief from pain, which might recur. True philosophy gives eternal peace and bliss. Vedanta does so.

Q.—What are the arguments to prove your position?

A.—Arguments are three—1, authority; 2, reason; 3, experience.

Q.—What is authority?

A.—Authority is the Veda, as interpreted by the light of Nature, Upaniṣads, and the sayings of the great men of different climes and ages.

APPENDIX I.

Q.—Quote some passages from the Veda, to prove the identity of human and divine spirits.

A.—Such passages of the Vedas are known as *mahárákyas*.
1. *Tat twam asi* :—Thou art that (*Brahma*).
2. *Ayam átma Brahma* :— This self (*Átma*) is Brahma.
3. *Ekamevadwitiyam* :—One without a second.
4. *Tasya bhasa sarvam idam bibhati* :—His light illumines all these.
5. *Yo sarasau Purushah soham asmi* :—What is this *purusha* (Brahma), the same am I.
6. *Dvitiad vai bhayam bhavati* :—From duality there is fear.
7. *Neha nánásti kinchana* :—All the appearances are nothing.
8. *Sarva khalvidam Brahma* :—All this is verily Brahma.

Q.—Give some other authorities from the teachings of other nations.

A.—1. Socrates said :—" The soul was allied to the Divine Being by similarity of nature."
2. Plato believed this world a mirage, non-reality, and an obstacle to divine knowledge.
3. Cicero said :—" I would swear that the soul is divine."
4. M. A. Antoninus says :—" Soul is all-intelligence, and a portion of the divinity."
5. Plotinus taught :—" By reducing the soul to abstraction we are one with the Infinite."
6. Philo says :—" The soul of man is divine."
7. Proclus :—" Know the divinity that is within you, that you may know the divine one, of which your soul is a ray."
8. Spinoza :—" God is the only substance."
9. Mansûr, a Muhammadam mystic, was crucified, because he said ' Anal Haq ' (I am God.)
10. Hafiz Shams-i-Tabriz, Mawlana Rumi, Abu Ali Kalendar, were all Vedantists. Christ said : " Ye are gods."

Q.—What are the reasons that the soul is divine and the world a dream ?

*A.—If we believe that the human soul is different from God, then the question arises in what relation does that God stand

---

*If we do not believe the soul to be a portion of divinity and the world a dream, we are forced to the other hypothesis that the soul is separate from God, and

to us? As a ruler, he would seem to be the most tyrannical being, seeing that the world is full of misery. But this need not be a stumbling block, if we believe that the whole world is a dream. We have many consciousnesses—our waking consciousness, our sleeping consciousness of *susupti*, our dreaming, and our divine consciousness. Now in every one of these states, the ideas presented to us seem to be real, and for the time being we believe them to be real. But no sooner is that state changed, than we think the ideas of that state to be unreal, and the ideas of our new state to be real. Therefore, the world is an idea, and spirit the only substance.

Q.—The dreams of no two persons ever coincide, nor do the same dreams recur again. If then the world were a dream, how do all men see it in the same way, and why does it always appear the same?

A.—The world is not a dream of an ordinary man ; the universe is a dream in the consciousness of the Brahma. As a great magnetiser can make his audience see, hear, perceive, &c., anything which he strongly wills, so the eternal will of the Brahma has made this world through his *Mâyâ* or willforce or delusion. He wills that we should see so and so, and we do so : but when we become He, the delusion vanishes.

Q.—If the world be a dream, there is no such thing as vice or virtue, good or bad, and we are not responsible for what we do.

A.—The world is false from *paramârthika* point of view, but is real from relative point of view, and for all practical purposes we must consider it to be so. As a cup of water will intoxicate a mesmerised subject, if he is told that it is wine, though water has no such property, so a person, as long as he is not emancipated, will suffer the consequences of his *karmas*, simply because he still is involved in *Mâyâ*.

---

the world is a reality. If these two substances—soul and Matter—be real, then they must be eternal, for to say that they were created by the will of God from nothing is an absurdity, for out of nothing something cannot be produced. To say that the substance of matter came out of God would also be derogatory to His dignity, for then non-intelligence would come out of perfect intelligence. For similar reasons, the materialistic theory, that soul is an evolution of matter is untenable, as, according to this doctrine intelligence would be produced out of non-intelligence. Thus we are led to three alternatives —(1) to believe the soul and matter to be eternal, which would be atheistic : it would do away with God ; (2) the substance of the world is a portion of God—a doctrine derogatory to Godhead ; (3) that the soul is a portion of divinity, and the world a dream.

APPENDIX I.

Q.—How do you prove from experience that Paramâtmâ and Jivâtmâ are one?

A.—Because the lives of those persons who had reached the threshold of Nirvâna prove it conclusively. They possessed all those attributes which we ascribe to God. They performed deeds which we in our ignorance call miracles and supernatural. Persons like Krishna, Buddha, Shankarâchârya show by their lives that they are gods.

Q.—How should one, then, practically unite himself with God?

A.—The method lies through the practice of Yoga.

Q.—Define Yoga.

A.—Yoga is the suspension of the various modifications of the mind.

Q.—How many kinds of Yoga are there?

A.—Many kinds of Yoga have been enumerated by ancient authors, i.e., Karma Yoga or Hatha Yoga, Mantra Yoga, Râja Yoga, &c. But of all these, only the Hatha Yoga and the Râja Yoga need be mentioned here.

Q.—Define and distinguish between the Hatha Yoga and the Râja Yoga.

A.—The Hatha Yoga is a process of physical training, in order to strengthen the will. The Râja Yoga is a process of pure mental training, for the same purpose. The Hatha Yoga is the lowest, the Râja Yoga the middle, and the Siva Yoga (i.e., spiritual method) the highest.

Q.—How should one practise Râja Yoga?

A.—The *adhikâri*, as defined above, should select first a suitable place, free from all disturbances, &c., and a suitable time when his mind is pure and elevated, and his body in its normal healthy state. He should practise *yama, niyama, âsana, prânâyâma, pratyâhara* and *sanyama*.

Q.—Define Yama.

A.—Yama is the first step of Yoga. It requires the *adhikâri* to practise the following five virtues:—

(1). *Ahinsâ*:—Not killing or doing injury to any animal, and not eating animal food.

(2). *Satya*:—Speaking truth under every circumstance.

(3). *Asteya*:—Non-stealing.

(4). *Bramacharya*:—Continence and chastity of mind and deed.

(5). *Aparigraha* :—Non-covetousness of things of this as well as of the world to come.

Q.—What is Niyama?

A.—The Niyama is also fivefold—

(1). *Saucha* :—Purification of body and mind.

(2). *Santoṣa* :—Contentment with one's state, without grumbling.

(3). *Tapas* :—Purification of bodily senses.

(4). *Swadhyâya* :--Silently muttering any religious formula, and study of sacred books.

(5). *Iswara pranidhâna* :—Persevering devotion to God.

Q.—What *âsana* (posture) should one adopt?

A.—Any posture which is steady and convenient. Do not change it at all.

Q.—What should one do after this?

A.—Having assumed a steady and pleasant posture, let him practise *prâṇâyâma*, *if he likes*. Prâṇâyâma is not absolutely necessary for Râja Yoga. The general method of Prâṇâyâma "consists in three modifications of breathing. The first act is expiration, which is performed through the right nostril, while the left is closed with the fingers of the right hand ; this is called *Rechaka* ; the thumb is then placed upon the right nostril and the fingers raised from the left, through which breath is inhaled ; this is called *Puraka* ; in the third act both nostrils are closed and breathing suspended ; this is *Kumbhaka*." First *Puraka*, then *Kumbhaka* and then *Rechaka*. The *Kumbhaka* or non-breathing should at least be practised for 30 seconds. To estimate this period, repeat last 30 times the mantra. When the practice of Prâṇâyâma becomes complete, Pratyâhâra will follow, *i.e.*, the practitioner will become insensible to all external things. He will not feel if one pinches his body ; he will not hear if you fire a gun near him, and so on. In Râja yoga you need not practise Prâṇâyâma, in order to bring about Pratyâhâra.

Q.—How should one practise Râja Yoga?

A.—The Râja Yoga may be divided into three parts—

(1). *Indriya-sanyama* :—Subjugation of the senses.

(2). *Mano-sanyama* :—Subjugation of the mind.

(3). *Laya* :—Absorption.

To attain *Indriya-sanyama* (*i.e.*, Pratyâhâra, you should strongly *imagine* that you are out of the body and moving in *âkâsa*.

APPENDIX I.

Practise for months till you attain the power of throwing your body into catalepsy whenever you like. It will be easier if you begin step by step, *e.g.*, *will* strongly that you will not *hear* any external sound, so much so that you should be able to make yourself deaf, whenever you like. This is hard of course, but not impossible, and requires patience. Having subdued the ear, try to subdue in a similar way the senses of sight, taste, smell, and touch. Having conquered the external senses, go to the internal senses, hunger, thirst, and conquer them too. Firm faith and persevering practice will bring about speedy success.

Q.— What is *Mano-sanyama?*

A.—One who has got mastery over his senses, to him the subjugation of mind is not very difficult. The first blow should be struck at memory and reasoning faculties. Then the association of ideas should be stopped, and so on. Thus the human soul which is pure consciousness, will be free from the trammels of senses and mind, and become *mukta*. When it has reached the *mukta* state, let it try to reach the *Laya* state, and plunging into the Divinity, become *one* with it. This will come last of all, and is known as *Kaivalyam*. But long before this state is attained, the Yogi will be amply rewarded for his toil by the attainment of psychic powers or *siddhis*. Even in the first stage, *i.e.*, of *Indriya-sanyama*, he will begin to see things at a distance clairvoyantly, and will perceive and read the thoughts of others. The whole secret of Yoga consists in making yourself a VOID, a VACUUM for the influx of Divinity. KNOW THYSELF is the secret of Philosophy, but VOID THYSELF is the secret of Nirvâna or Divine Wisdom.

APPENDIX II.

AN ACCOUNT OF SÂDHU HARIDAS.

It was in the year 1839 that I had returned to Lahore, after having visited the European continent and my native country. I enjoyed the pleasure, on my return, of being the companion of General Ventura, who was also hastening to India to resume his duties. On our voyage, we had many conversations, among which, the events which had happened during my absence from Lahore underwent discussion. On that occasion, the General related to me an occurrence which, at first, I could scarcely believe, thinking it a pure invention or a mere joke; but I soon became persuaded that he was in earnest. I give it here with the remark only, that, after having arrived at Lahore, I heard it confirmed by other persons, in whose statements I could also place confidence.

Runjeet Sing—thus runs the narrative—was told that a saat, or faqueer, living in the mountains, was able to keep himself in a state resembling death, and would allow himself to be even buried, without injuring or endangering his life, provided they would remove or release him from the grave after expiration of a fixed time, he being in the possession of the means of resuscitating himself again. The Maharajah thought it impossible. To convince himself of the truth of the assertion, he ordered the faqueer to be brought to his court, and caused him to undergo the experiment, assuring him that no precaution would be omitted to discover whether it was a deception. In consequence, the faqueer, in the presence of the court, placed himself in a complete state of *asphyxia*, having all the appearance of death.

In that state, he was wrapped in the linen on which he was sitting, the seal of Runjeet Sing was stamped thereon, and it was placed in a chest, on which the Maharajah put a strong lock. The chest was buried in a garden, outside the city, belonging to to the minister, barley was sown on the ground, and the space enclosed with a wall and surrounded by sentinels. On the fortieth day, which was the time fixed for his exhumation, a great number of the authorities of the durbar, with General Ventura, and several Englishmen from the vicinity, one of them a medical man,

APPENDIX II.

went to the enclosure. The chest was brought up and opened, and the faqueer was found in the same position as they had left him, cold and stiff. A friend of mine told me that had I been present when they endeavoured to bring him to life, by applying warmth to the head, injecting air into his ears and mouth, and rubbing the whole of his body to promote circulation, &c., I should certainly not have had the slightest doubt of the reality of the performance. The minister, Rajah Dhyan Sing, assured me, that he himself kept this faqueer (whose name was Haridas) four months under the ground, when he was at Jummoo in the mountains. On the day of his burial, he ordered his beard to be shaved, and at his exhumation his chin was as smooth as on the day of his interment, thus furnishing a complete proof of the powers of vitality having been suspended during that period. He likewise caused himself to be interred at Jesrota, in the mountains, and at Umritsir, and also by the English in Hindostan. In the *Calcutta Medical Journal*, about 1835, there is a full description of the faqueer, and we are there informed, that he preferred having the chest, in which he was enclosed, suspended in the air, instead of its being buried beneath the earth, as he feared the possibility of his body being attacked by ants, whilst in that middle state between life and death. Having, however, refused to undergo another trial, several of the English people there doubted the truth of the story, and refused credence is so astonishing a power.* But it is quite certain that had there been any deception as regards the interment of the faqueer, rendering his experiment easy of accomplishment, those engaged or associated with him, and to whom the task of restoring the vital energies was necessarily entrusted, would, of necessity, be acquainted with the mystery, and be able, since his real decease, to emulate his example; that, however, is not the case. It appears, consequently, that the faqueer was the only one then in possession of that power; and, as a further corroboration of this view of the case, I may mention that I myself inquired in the Panjab, in the mountains and valleys of Cashmere, and in other parts of India, and made every exertion to find a person possessed of this power, in order to take him to Europe, or at least to Calcutta, but without success. Several

---

* To corroborate the above, my readers can refer to General Ventura (Paris) and also the Colonel Sir C. M. Wade (London), who were present, and assisted at the restoration of the faqueer, some accounts of whom have been published from the Colonel's statement.

Hindoos told me that such faqueers set no value upon money; I replied to them, however, that, at all events, they fully appreciated other worldly pleasures. They did not like to hear this statement, implying that the faqueer was a *debauchee*. Several complaints had, however, been made of him, on which account Runjeet Sing intended to banish him from Lahore. He anticipated the intention, by eloping with a Khatrani (woman of a Hindoo caste) to the mountains, where he died, and was burned according to the custom of the country. His elopement with this woman may serve as a proof (in contradiction to other statements) that he was neither an eunuch nor a hermaphrodite.

Doubtless, it is a difficult task, and not within the power of every one, to acquire the skill necessary for the performance of this experiment, and those who do succeed must undergo a long and continual practice of preparatory measures. I was informed that such people have their *frœnulum linguæ* cut and entirely loosened, and that they get their tongue prominent, drawing and lengthening it by means of rubbing it with butter mixed with some pellitory of Spain, in order that they may be able to lay back the tongue at the time they are about to stop respiration, so as to cover the orifice of the hinder part of the *fosses nasales*, and thus (with other means for the same purpose, which I shall mention) keep the air shut up in the body and head.* Novices, in trying the experiment, shut their eyes, and press them with their fingers, as also the cavities of the ears and nostrils, because the natural warmth of the body might cause such an expansion of the enclosed gas as otherwise to produce, by the violence of its pressure, a rupture of some of those delicate organs not yet accustomed by practice to endure it. This, I am told, is especially the case with the eyes and the tympanum of the ear. For the better acquisition of this power, they are accustomed to practise the holding of the breath for a long period. They swallow a small strip of linen, in order to cleanse the stomach, and by a tube draw a quantity of water through the anus into the intestines to rinse them. This is performed while sitting in a vessel filled with water to the height of the arm-pits. It is said that the faqueer in question, a few days previous to his experiments, took some kind of purgative, and subsisted for several days on a coarse milk regimen. On the day of his

---

* A similar process is explained in some of the *Encyclopædias*, in the article on "Engastrimythe," or the mechanism of the ventriloquists.

burial, instead of food, he slowly swallowed, in the presence of the assembly, a rag of three fingers in breadth and thirty yards in length, and afterwards extracted it, for the purpose of removing all foreign matters from the stomach, having previously rinsed the bowels in the manner I have before mentioned. Ridiculous as this operation may appear to the reader, and as it appears, indeed, to me also, yet these artists must, of necessity, be complete masters of their body and its organism, and possess a more than ordinary power over the muscles. We are scarcely capable of swallowing a somewhat long piece of maccaroni if it is not well boiled and moistened with butter, &c., to render it palatable. It is probable, however, that they may have lost the sense of taste, and their neck-muscles may be relaxed to such a degree that the long linen strip does not meet with any resistance in the throat. These preparations being made, the faqueer stopped all the natural openings of the body with plugs of aromatic wax, placed back his tongue in the manner I have before indicated, crossed his arms over his breast, and thus suffocated himself, in the presence of a multitude of spectators. On his exhumation, one of the first operations is to draw his tongue into its natural position; after this, a warm aromatic paste, made from pulse meal, is placed on his head, and air is injected into his lungs and also through the ears, from which the plugs are withdrawn. By this operation, the pellets in the nostrils are driven out with considerable force and noise, and this is considered the first symptom of his resuscitation. Friction is then strenuously applied all over the body, and at length he begins to breathe naturally, opens his eyes, and is gradually restored to consciousness. It is related that, two hundred and fifty years ago, in the time of the Gooroo Arjun Sing, a Jogee faqueer was found in his tomb in a sitting posture, at Umritsir, and was restored to life. This faqueer is reported to have been below the ground for one hundred years; and when he revived, he related many circumstances connected with the times in which he had lived. Whether this tradition be true or false, it is impossible to say; but I am of opinion, that he, who can pass four months below the ground without becoming a prey to corruption, may also remain there for one year. Granting this, it is impossible to fix a limit to the time during which a suspension of the vital functions may continue, without injury to their subsequent power.

However paradoxical or absurd this statement may appear, and however persuaded I may be that many a reader, believing himself to be a wise man, will smile at the relation, I cannot, nevertheless, avoid confessing freely, that I do not entirely reject all the details given respecting the circumstances, for as Haller observes :—" In the interior of nature, no mortal can penetrate ; happy is he who knows a small part, even of its surface." We find much credence given to such phenomena in the most ancient traditions. Who will not remember the history of Epimenides of Creta, who, after a sleep of forty years in a grotto there, is reported to have again re-entered the world, from which he had so long been separated ! Who will not remember also the seven holy sleepers, who, according to a Vatican manuscript, were concealed in a grotto near Ephesus, in order to escape the persecutions of the Christians, during the reign of the Emperor Dacius, and who, 155 years subsequently, in the time of Theodosius II, returned to consciousness ? But even rejecting these traditions, have we not also similar examples in the animal kingdom ? Have not animals, especially toads, been detected in rocks, wherein, according to the calculations made, they had been enclosed for several centuries, in a state of sleep or torpor, and which animals, after having been brought into the air, have recovered their vitality ; and it is not necessary to remind the naturalist of the fact, that many species of animals invariably pass the winter season in a kind of sleep, awaking in the spring with renewed and unimpaired energies. Among recent cases, which demonstrate the great endurance of human life, is the following relation :—At Vienna, some years ago, a Hungarian was, during a period of twelve months, in a comatose state, and his jaw-bones were so firmly closed that it was impossible to open his mouth ; the physicians were consequently obliged to extract some of his teeth, in order to administer some remedies and broth, to preserve life ; he, nevertheless, at last recovered.

In the *Philosophical Transactions* for 1705 (Nov. and Dec., Vol. XVII, p. 2177), the history of a case is related, which supports what has been previously mentioned :—" A man of about twenty-five years of age, living in the neighbourhood of Bath, fell suddenly asleep, and continued for nearly a month in that state. Two years afterwards, he was again in a similar condition : his jaw-bones closed themselves ; he was unable to eat, but fell asleep, and continued to be devoid of sensation for seventeen weeks. This occurred at the time when barley was being sown, and when he again awoke it was quite ripe. In the month of August, he again fell asleep. He was bled; stimulating remedies were employed; and every means of restoration was used which the medical skill of the period could suggest, but in vain; he did not awake until the month of November." In Plott's Natural History of Oxfordshire (c. 8, sec. 11, p. 196, published in 1677), a case is alluded to, which, not being generally known, I will quote here, it being another evidence of the length of time during which a person may exist without nourishment.

"Rebekah Smith, the servant-maid of one Thomas White, of Minster Lovel, being above fifty years of age, and of a robust constitution, though she seldom ate flesh (it scarcely agreeing with her), after she came from the communion on Palm-Sunday, April 16, 1671, was taken with such a dryness in her throat, that she could not swallow her spittle, nor any thing else to supply the demands of nature; and in this state she continued, without eating or drinking, to the amazement of all, for about *ten weeks*, viz., to the 29th of June, being both St. Peter's and Witney fair day; by which time, being brought very low, her master made inquiry, and found out a person who gave him an amulet (for, it was supposed, she was bewitched) against this evil; after the application of this amulet, within two or three days (though I dare not suppose there was any connection between the medicine and the disease), she first drank a little water, then warm broths in small quantities at a time, and nothing else till Palm-Sunday again, twelve months after, when she began to eat bread and other food as she had formerly done; and the record states that she was then about the age of sixty, and still living in the same place, ready to testify to the truth of the matter; as were also Thomas White and his wife, who were the only other persons living in the house with her, and who would confidently assert (for they carefully observed), that they did not believe she ever took anything whatever in those *ten weeks* time, nor anything more than what is before mentioned until the expiration of the year."

The London Medical and Physical Journal, Vol. XXXV, p. 509, states that:—

"An account of the sleeping woman of Dunnibald, near Montrose, was read by the Rev. James Brewster, at the

Royal Society of Edinburgh. Her first sleeping fit lasted from the 27th to the 30th of June, 1815. Next morning she again fell into a sleep which lasted seven days, without motion, food, or evacuation. At the end of this time, by moving her hand and pointing to her mouth, it was understood she wanted food, which was given to her; but she remained in her lethargic state till the 8th of August, six weeks in all, without appearing to be awake, except on the 30th of June," &c., &c. This case is well authenticated.

And in J. N. Willan's Miscellaneous Work, published by A. Smith, M. D., p. 339, he states that he had seen many, mostly Jews and other aliens, of a dark, swarthy complexion, sometimes lie six or eight weeks in the torpid, insensible condition above described.—*Honnigberger's " Thirty-five years in the East."*